P9-DVQ-030

APRIL 4

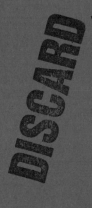
DISCARD

SLEEP RIGHT IN FIVE NIGHTS

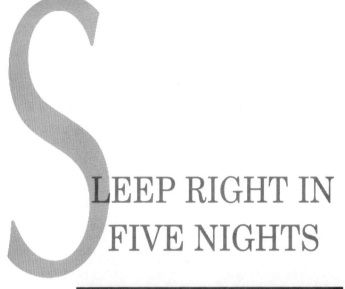

SLEEP RIGHT IN FIVE NIGHTS

A Clear and Effective Guide for Conquering Insomnia

James Perl, Ph.D.

William Morrow and Company, Inc.
New York

Library of Congress Cataloging-in-Publication Data

Perl, James.
    Sleep right in five nights : a clear and effective guide for conquering
  insomnia / James Perl.
      p. cm.
    ISBN 0-688-12248-5
    1. Insomnia—Popular works. 2. Insomnia—Treatment.   I. Title.
  RC548.P47 1993
  616.8'498—dc20   93-16379
                                                                 CIP

Printed in the United States of America

First Edition

1   2   3   4   5   6   7   8   9   10

BOOK DESIGN BY LISA STOKES

*This book is dedicated to the life and memory
of my father, Oscar Perl (1916–1986).*

Acknowledgments

MANY SLEEP RESEARCHERS HAVE WORKED TO DEVELOP OUR understanding of sleep and ways to improve it. I acknowledge my debt to those scientists, whose ideas and research findings form the foundation of this book.

I am particularly indebted to Mayo Clinic psychologist Peter Hauri, a pioneer in the research and treatment of insomnia. His contributions have added much to the field of sleep disorders and to this book.

I am grateful to these sleep researchers who generously shared their expertise by commenting on portions of this book as it was being prepared:

Richard Bootzin, Ph.D.
University of Arizona

Thomas Coates, Ph.D.
University of California

8   Acknowledgments

William Dement, M.D., Ph.D.
Stanford University

Peter Hauri, Ph.D.
Mayo Clinic
Rochester, Minnesota

J. Allan Hobson, M.D.
Harvard University

James Horne, Ph.D.
Loughborough University
Leicestershire, England

Reese Jones, M.D.
University of California

Patricia Lacks, Ph.D.
Washington University
St. Louis, Missouri

Alfred Lewy, M.D., Ph.D.
University of Oregon

David Minors, Ph.D.
University of Manchester
Manchester, England

Arthur Spielman, Ph.D.
City University of New York

Carl Thoresen, Ph.D.
Stanford University

James Waterhouse, Ph.D.
University of Manchester
Manchester, England

I also thank these experts in fields related to sleep who reviewed and commented on sections of the manuscript:

Michael Anziano, Ph.D.
Fort Lewis College
Durango, Colorado

James Ascough, Ph.D.
Wabash Valley Mental Health Center
West Lafayette, Indiana

Kathleen Curran
Four Corners Yoga
Hesperus, Colorado

Albert Ellis, Ph.D.
Institute for Rational-Emotive Therapy
New York, New York

Stephen Hodge, Ph.D.
University of Colorado

Louis Lemberger, Ph.D., M.D.
Indiana University

Peter Lewinsohn, Ph.D.
Oregon Research Institute
Eugene, Oregon

Laura Moore, R. Ph.
Rocky Mountain Drug Consultation Center
Denver, Colorado

Wilse Webb, Ph.D.
University of Florida

Barton Schmitt, M.D.
University of Colorado

Wilse Webb, Ph.D.
University of Florida

Andrew Weil, M.D.
University of Arizona

I appreciate the help of Tom Cordas, director of the sleep disorders center at Presbyterian/St. Luke's Medical Center in Denver.
Vance Aandahl reviewed the manuscript and offered

many strong suggestions. At William Morrow and Company, Nancy Gallt and Pearl Hanig were very helpful. My editor, Andy Dutter, provided guidance and made the publication process a pleasure.

I am grateful to my wife, K.K. DuVivier, who suggested that I write this book. Her editing and her support were invaluable throughout the project.

Finally, I am indebted to the insomnia sufferers who shared with me their concerns, frustrations, successes, and insights about sleep.

Contents

12   Contents

14 Contents

Contents   17

Introduction to the Reader:
What This Book Will Do for You

YOU TURN OFF THE LIGHT AT BEDTIME, BUT YOU CAN'T TURN off your mind as the bedside clock ticks off the minutes one by one. Or you awaken at 3:00 A.M. and lie there wondering if you'll still be awake when the alarm goes off.

Maybe your job was particularly stressful today, and you can't stop thinking about work. It might be a night when you really want to sleep well, before tomorrow's big meeting. Or it could be that nothing is bothering you — except for the fact that you can't sleep.

If this scene seems familiar to you, be assured that you have a lot of company. Approximately one-third of all American adults have had insomnia during the previous year, and half of this group reports severe or constant sleep problems.

Nearly all of us experience sleeplessness at one time or another. Unlike some problems we grow out of, insomnia remains with many of us throughout life, changing only in its intensity and its particular form. College students sleep on a different schedule each night, then find that they can't fall asleep the night before a big exam. Job-related anxieties, family stresses, and medical conditions can disrupt sleep at any age. Older adults don't seem to sleep as deeply as they used to, or they awaken long before dawn, unable to get back to sleep at all.

If you have tried over-the-counter sleep medication, you may have found that it gave relief for a few weeks, then lost effectiveness. You may have tried psychotherapy or counting sheep. For most people, those attempts to solve a sleep problem don't make a lasting difference.

But help is now available for insomnia sufferers. Highly effective techniques to improve nighttime sleep — and daytime wakefulness — have been developed during the past two decades. More than two thousand members of the American Sleep Disorders Association engage in research and practice at universities, sleep disorders centers, and other places around the nation. Scientists and clinicians are also at work worldwide, especially in Europe and Japan. These physicians, psychologists, and other professionals are using techniques that have helped thousands of insomnia sufferers sleep better.

Modern methods have been proved effective in overcoming insomnia, and improvements in sleep quality have been shown to last for years. *Sleep Right in Five Nights* summarizes the most useful techniques developed by sleep researchers and clinicians, in a program that brings relief to most insomnia sufferers in just five nights.

The two chapters in Part I contain important information you need to know about sleep and sleep problems. In Part II you will find a step-by-step guide to help you diagnose the cause of your insomnia. You'll learn a lot about insomnia as you complete the diagnostic questionnaire. An optional sleep log can help you confirm the hunches about the cause of your insomnia that you came up with in the questionnaire. But you can follow the book's program even if you don't complete the sleep log.

After reading the diagnostic chapters of Part II, you probably will have a good idea of what's causing your sleep problem. Based on what you learned, you will read one or more corresponding chapters in Part III. These eight chapters survey the major causes of insomnia and what to do about them. You will see how sleep and sleep problems change with normal aging. You will learn how sleep is affected by medical conditions, medications, sleeping pills, caffeine, tobacco, and alcohol. You will find out how stress, anxiety, and depression can cause sleeplessness. You will learn how disruptions of the body's sleep-wake rhythms can lead to Sunday-night insomnia and other sleep problems. And you will see how you can unwittingly learn to associate your bed and bedroom with wakefulness rather than with sleep. For each of these causes, Part III presents the most effective solution.

The best way to overcome insomnia is to identify its cause and take action to change it. But some people can't figure out why they don't sleep well. The four chapters of Part IV will help you whether or not you know the cause of your insomnia. You will learn guidelines for napping, nutrition, exercise, and evening routines to court sleep. You will learn how to prevent worrying in bed. You will learn sleep-inducing bedtime relaxation exercises and mind games. A single idea from these chapters that works for you can make a big difference in the quality of your sleep. The techniques are easy to learn and easy to use. The only investment they require is a little time.

In the book's final chapter you will find out about the Sleep CURE, a program that improves sleep for nearly all insomnia sufferers, whether the problem is falling asleep, staying asleep, or both.

The Epilogue will show you how to maintain good sleep habits over the years and what to do when progress doesn't come easily. Appendices present detailed scripts for the most effective types of sleep-inducing relaxation instructions. Other appendices examine shift work, jet lag, children's sleep problems, and sleep disorders centers.

Whether your sleep problem comes and goes, or whether you suffer from insomnia nearly every night, this book will help you. You will begin to get relief from sleeplessness in just five nights. You will learn skills for falling asleep and staying asleep. And you will take control of your sleep for the rest of your life.

Part I
Sleep and Sleep Problems

THE TWO CHAPTERS OF PART I WILL GIVE YOU BACKGROUND information that is helpful for understanding and solving your sleep problem.

Chapter 1 presents the facts about sleep that are most relevant to insomnia sufferers. This chapter will help you sort the truth from the many common misconceptions about sleep. You will gain understanding about basic sleep processes and how they relate to insomnia and other sleep problems.

Chapter 2 surveys the many different kinds of sleep disorders. You will learn about the most common sleep problem — insomnia — and its causes. In addition, you will learn about other types of sleep disorders that sometimes accompany insomnia.

Reading the facts about sleep in Part I will help you make the best use of the information in the remainder of the book.

1

What You Need to Know About Sleep

IT IS IMPORTANT TO KNOW A FEW BASIC FACTS ABOUT SLEEP before we examine insomnia and how to cure it. Let's begin by considering several important issues about sleep and insomnia:

- *How much sleep you need*
- *The consequences of losing sleep*
- *Making up lost sleep*
- *What happens during sleep*
- *Changes in sleep as you grow older*
- *Why some people sleep better than others*

Much common folklore about sleep is based on inaccurate notions. This chapter will help you sift the facts from fiction.

HOW MUCH SLEEP YOU NEED

The average length of sleep is about seven and a half hours for young adults and seven hours for people in late middle age. But this is like saying that the typical person wears a size seven or seven and a half shoe. The average does not begin to reflect the wide range of individual differences.

About two-thirds of adults sleep between six and nine hours per night. The other third sleep more or less than this range. Genetic variation accounts for the wide range in the amount of sleep we each need. That is, our individual sleep needs are largely programmed at birth by hereditary factors.

People's need for sleep depends in part on their emotional state and the level of stress they are experiencing. People in a particularly happy period may need less sleep than usual. During times of stress or depression, people often change their sleep habits: Some get more sleep than usual; others get less. Some women need additional sleep during their premenstrual periods.

Sleep specialists describe people who sleep less than six hours as *short sleepers*. One of every five adults is a short sleeper. For example, Thomas Edison slept four or five hours a night. Documented reports of individuals needing just three hours of sleep are common in the professional literature, and scientists have studied well-functioning people who have slept between forty minutes and one hour a night throughout their entire adult lives. Slightly more men than women are short sleepers.

Many people believe the myth that everyone needs eight hours of sleep a night. Some worry needlessly because they sleep less than this standard. If you are reading this book because you sleep less than everyone else you know, you may not have an insomnia problem: You may just be a short sleeper. The way to know if you are sleeping enough is by evaluating your daytime alertness and energy level. If you feel wide-awake, alert, and energetic throughout the day, you are getting enough sleep at night. Trying to sleep more is likely to create an insomnia problem for yourself.

At the opposite extreme, people who sleep more than nine hours are considered *long sleepers*. One in ten adults is a long sleeper. For example, Albert Einstein — like many creative people — needed at least ten hours of sleep each night. Slightly more women than men are long sleepers.

When the sleeping patterns of short sleepers and long sleepers are compared, one major difference emerges. Short sleepers spend a larger proportion of sleep time in the deep sleep that refreshes and revitalizes the body. Short sleepers sleep more efficiently than long sleepers.

Some researchers have claimed that there are differences in personality between short and long sleepers. Short sleepers have been thought to be energetic, confident, ambitious, and successful; in contrast, long sleepers have been described as lethargic, passive underachievers. However, other researchers dispute these claims regarding personality differences between the two groups. The only clear conclusion appears to be that extreme short sleepers — those who sleep less than four and a half hours a night — are more energetic than others.

Bed partners often have sleep requirements that differ greatly. Problems may arise if one person expects the other to conform to a certain sleep pattern, because the amount of sleep we need is largely hereditary — that is, determined by individual genetic factors.

The most effective way for a couple to cope with a situation in which one person needs more sleep than the other is to try to agree on a mutual bedtime or a mutual waking time. That is, if both partners go to bed at the same time, the short sleeper will need to get up earlier. Alternatively, both can awaken at the same time if the short sleeper goes to bed later than the partner.

Consider the case of Mr. Stanton, a man in his twenties who sought counseling for what he thought was an insomnia problem involving trouble falling asleep. Each night he and his wife went to bed around 10:30. On most nights she fell asleep promptly, but he lay in bed tossing and turning. He might get up and read or watch television until finally he fell asleep sometime between midnight and 1:30 A.M. In the morning he and his wife both got up at 6:00. Although he usually got around five hours of sleep, Mr. Stanton always awoke refreshed and remained alert throughout the day. Yet he and his wife were convinced that there was something wrong because he didn't sleep as long as she.

Mr. Stanton learned that instead of having an insomnia problem, he was merely a short sleeper. He began going to bed later than his wife, so that they both could get up at the same time. Although he continued to spend much of his late-night time watching television and reading, he was relieved to learn that there was nothing wrong with his ability to sleep.

You can conduct your own simple research study to determine how much sleep you really need. Begin by figuring out your average nightly sleep length. Then do either of two experiments. If you feel alert and rested during the day with your regular sleep length, try sleeping an hour less. If the change makes you sleepy during the day, return to the longer amount of sleep you had been getting. But if you feel alert and rested with this shorter amount, you can continue with the reduced night's sleep.

If you feel sleepy during the day with your current amount of nightly sleep, you can conduct a different experiment. After you initially figure out your average nightly sleep length, schedule one *more* hour of sleep each night. If you feel more alert during the day with this longer amount, you should continue sleeping longer. If more sleep doesn't improve your daytime tiredness, review the different disorders surveyed in Chapter 2. One of them may be causing your daytime sleepiness.

Whether you experiment by reducing or increasing your sleep time, carry on the experiment for about a week because it can take your body that long to adapt to a new sleep length. Continue to adjust your sleep time down or up, until you find what seems to be a good balance. Don't worry about getting eight hours or any other standard. Instead sleep the amount that feels right for you.

THE CONSEQUENCES OF LOSING SLEEP

You probably know what it feels like to lose a lot of sleep over a period of several days. You have little energy and little motivation. You feel listless and drowsy. You lack spontaneity and go through the day grimly serious. Accomplishing your work seems burdensome and takes great effort. You feel depleted, with no reserves to draw on.

That's the bad news about the effects of losing sleep. There is good news as well.

Most people assume that loss of sleep causes their mental and motor abilities to decline. The belief that we won't be able to perform well the next day often contributes to our distress — and to our insomnia — during a sleepless night. However, a large body of research on sleep deprivation shows that performance suffers significantly only after about sixty hours of lost sleep.

In sleep-restriction experiments, subjects who normally sleep seven to eight hours are asked to sleep smaller amounts. These studies show that the human body has a remarkable tolerance for sleep loss. Only three behavioral effects of sleep deprivation are consistently observed:

1. Subjects report daytime drowsiness, especially during sedentary activities.
2. Subjects tend to become a bit grouchy and irritable.
3. Performance drops slightly on routine or boring clerical tasks — for example, adding columns of numbers. Performance on more complex tasks typically is un-

affected. However, some subjects have difficulty producing highly creative work.

These three effects are the only significant consequences of losing sleep. And even they subside within one or two weeks, as subjects become accustomed to sleeping less.

We can function well the day after a poor night's sleep because we complete all of our most restorative sleep in the first three to five hours. After that we are in shallower stages of sleep, not far from wakefulness. (We will examine the different sleep stages later in this chapter.)

Losing even an entire night of sleep will not make a big difference the next day. Typically you will feel most sleepy around 3:00 or 4:00 A.M. But if you remain awake, you will get a second wind by 8:00 or 9:00 A.M., and you will function fine throughout the day.

In one experiment, four men were kept awake for over eight days with no ill effects. In another instance of extreme sleep deprivation, a high-school student broke the world record in 1965 for sustained wakefulness. He remained awake for 264 hours, or eleven days. During this period he was carefully observed by members of the Stanford University Sleep Disorders Center. He became somewhat irritable and had difficulty concentrating after the fourth day, but his performance on mental and motor tasks did not decline significantly.

So we can function well even when we lose sleep. But what about our health? Many people think that sleep loss causes serious health problems. For example, about half the respondents in one survey inaccurately believed that chronic sleep loss can contribute to heart attacks. However, the only apparent health consequence of sleep loss concerns the body's defenses against viral disease. Research presented at the 1993 annual conference of the World Federation of Sleep Society shows that losing three hours or more of sleep can decrease the efficiency of the immune system by as much as 50 percent. So there is some truth in the notion that sleep helps us ward off sickness. But the immune system returns to normal when you begin getting more sleep. On the day after you've lost a lot of sleep, be especially aware of situations with potential exposure to viruses.

Physicians Ian Oswald and Kirstine Adam, of the Sleep Research Laboratory at Edinburgh University in Scotland, review research on health effects of sleep loss in their book *Get a Better Night's Sleep* (New York: Arco Publishing, 1983). They conclude: "We must emphasize that you cannot die of loss of sleep, nor will you suffer long-term mental or physical ill-effects as a result. You can take comfort from the fact that sleep is a self-regulating system so that when we really need it, we get it and almost nothing will stop us."

The mistaken belief that losing sleep is harmful can cause anxiety about sleep loss. This anxiety can make it harder to fall asleep. Difficulty falling asleep can further increase anxiety, and this increased anxiety can interfere even more with sleep, and so on. However, knowing the truth — that sleep loss does not hurt you — will help you break this cycle of insomnia and worry about insomnia. The facts are reassuring.

CAN YOU MAKE UP LOST SLEEP? AND DO YOU HAVE TO?

You don't need to repay your sleep debt on an hour-for-hour basis. People deprived of sleep for days don't sleep around the clock to make up the sleep they lost. For example, the student who stayed awake for eleven days didn't need to sleep eighty or ninety hours afterward. Instead he slept fourteen and a half hours, then resumed sleeping his normal eight-hour nights with no apparent mental or physical aftereffects.

We can make up lost sleep efficiently because recovery sleep following sleep deprivation is deeper and of higher quality than usual. This fact should console any insomnia sufferer who has feared it will take a long time to recover from a bad night of sleep.

WHAT HAPPENS DURING SLEEP

Sleep encompasses about one-third of our existence; if it all occurred sequentially, it would fill twenty-five years of the average lifetime. Every night we experience the curious changes in consciousness called sleep. Yet this integral part of our lives is a dark mystery to most of us.

As recently as 1935, scientists thought sleep was a static, constant time of quiet inactivity. In that year, it was found that electrical charges emitted by the brain follow a regular progression during sleep. Now it is known that human sleep is a dynamic behavioral state made up of different levels of detachment from the world. During sleep, complex physical changes occur in our brains and throughout our bodies. As we sleep, our brain and body systems follow oscillating cycles. These cycles wax and wane regularly, along with the depth of sleep and the presence or absence of dream activity.

STAGES OF SLEEP

During the night your sleep progresses through four to six sleep cycles. A sleep cycle contains up to four sleep levels — or stages — each deeper than the one before. In addition, each sleep cycle contains a stage in which you dream. Let's see what happens during the stages of the night's first sleep cycle.

You enter the first stage of the night's first sleep cycle as soon as you fall asleep. Entering this stage is like descending a series of gradual steps.

Figure 1 depicts the different sleep cycles and their stages for children, young adults, and the elderly. The first cycle begins with Stage 1 sleep. This transition from wakefulness to the deeper stages of sleep lasts anywhere from thirty

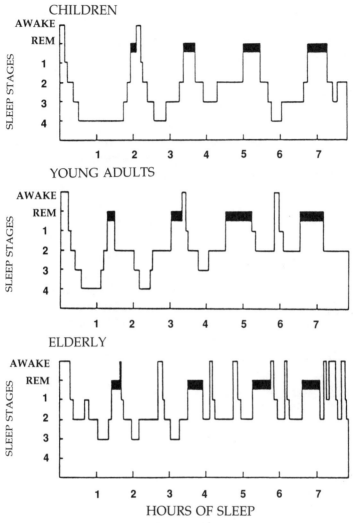

Figure 1–1

Sleep Cycles Across the Night at Three Age Levels

REM sleep (darkened area) occurs cyclically at intervals of about ninety minutes in all age-groups. Stage 4 sleep decreases progressively with age, so that little or none is present in the elderly. In addition, the elderly experience frequent awakenings and a signficant increase in time awake after sleep onset. From *Evaluation and Treatment of Insomnia* by Anthony Kales and Joyce Kales. Copyright ©1984. Reprinted by permission of Oxford University Press, Inc.

seconds to ten minutes. During stage 1 sleep, short dream-like experiences sometimes occur as thoughts drift off. However, these are not true dreams, as we will see later in this chapter.

In stage 1 sleep, body temperature begins to drop and the muscles become relaxed. But sleepers can be awakened easily from stage 1 sleep, and if aroused at this stage, people are often unaware that they have been sleeping at all.

After the very light sleep of stage 1 the sleeper enters the light-to-medium sleep of stage 2, which lasts thirty to forty-five minutes. During this time the sleeper can still be awakened readily. Sleepers spend more time in stage 2 than in any other stage — approximately half the night's sleep. Stage 2 sleep is of moderate value in restoring the body.

The sleeper progresses from stage 2 to the deep sleep of stages 3 and 4. As one stage blends into the next, breathing and muscles become more relaxed, heart rate slows, and sensitivity to sound and light diminishes. The sleeper becomes much more difficult to awaken.

Sleep is measured primarily through an *electroencephalogram*—from the Greek *electro* (electrical), *encephalon* (brain), *gram* (written record) — or EEG. There is more about the measurement of sleep on page 312 in the section on sleep disorders centers.

The EEG of stages 3 and 4 sleep is characterized by *delta waves*, a slow brain-wave pattern that accompanies the quiet brain of deep sleep. Stages 3 and 4 differ from each other only in the amount of delta waves each contains. Fewer than half of the brain waves in stage 3 sleep are delta, and half or more of the brain waves in stage 4 sleep are delta. Because delta waves characterize stages 3 and 4 sleep, these two stages are sometimes called *delta sleep*.

Stages 3 and 4 are of most value in restoring and revitalizing the body. A sleeper deprived of the deep sleep in stages 3 and 4 will awaken feeling unrefreshed.

The length of deep sleep is shortened by alcohol and by

some psychoactive medications, as later chapters show. In Part IV we will examine ways to increase the proportion of deep sleep you get at night.

REM Sleep

Following stage 4, your sleep becomes shallower as you ascend the steps you went down when you first fell asleep. You return to stage 3, then stage 2. Then, instead of ascending through stage 1 to wakefulness, you enter the night's first period of dream sleep.

When we dream, our eyes move quickly back and forth. For this reason the stage of sleep during which we dream is called *REM sleep*. REM is an acronym for *rapid eye movement*. (Most sleep, stages 1 through 4, is simply called non-REM sleep.) It is not known with certainty whether eye movements mean that we are actually "watching" actions in our dreams. However, many experts believe that during dreams our eyes move to correspond with the dream's actions.

During REM sleep our brain activity resembles the pattern that occurs during wakefulness. Our heart rate increases to its waking level. Men experience penile erections; women undergo clitoral erections and increased blood flow to the vaginal area. These sexual reactions usually are unrelated to dream content; instead they reflect the body's general physiological arousal during REM sleep.

REM sleep occupies about one-fourth of the night. This stage occurs on average every ninety minutes. REM periods become progressively longer as sleep progresses, and most REM sleep occurs in the second half of the night. The night's first dream lasts only about five minutes. Dreams during the next two intervals last about ten and fifteen minutes respectively. By the time of the fourth interval, dream sequences last thirty minutes to an hour. We forget nearly all our dreams except those that occur right before we awaken.

The most plausible explanation for the meaning of

dreams is the *activation-synthesis theory*, proposed by Harvard psychiatrists and neurophysiologists J. Allan Hobson and Robert McCarley. Simply stated, this theory holds that dreaming is the incidental outcome of physiological brain activity during sleep.

The oldest and most primitive part of our brain is the brainstem. This area, at the base of the brain, is an enlargement of the spinal cord. The brainstem, which is sometimes called the *lower brain,* controls such basic bodily functions as respiration and temperature regulation. About every ninety minutes, during REM sleep, the brainstem spontaneously generates random bursts of nerve-cell activity. This intense neurological activity travels from the primitive lower brain to the cerebral cortex — sometimes called the *upper brain* — the center of sensation and thought. The lower brain's neurological noise activates the upper brain.

According to the activation-synthesis theory, dreams are the result of the upper brain's attempts to make sense of this random neurological bombardment. The cerebral cortex organizes the nerve-cell activity through a synthesis that includes memories, feelings, and current preoccupations.

Dream content often relates to the person's thoughts and actions before sleep. Research has shown that when people watch horror films before bedtime, they usually dream about the content of the films. To prevent troubling dreams, it is best to avoid anxious thoughts or stressful activities before you go to bed. We will return to this point in Chapter 14.

The brain seems not to realize that the body is asleep during REM. It gives commands to the muscles to engage in the actions portrayed in the dream, as if the person were awake. However, these actions are not carried out, because just before the dream period a group of nerve cells in the lower brain immobilizes all of the body's large muscles (smaller muscles may move occasionally). Because the body's large muscles are immobilized, REM sleep is a semiparalyzed state in which the brain's commands to move muscles produce only slight twitches. You may have noticed these twitches, like inhibited running movements, in dreaming dogs or cats.

During deep sleep most of the body's blood is directed to the muscles. This blood flow facilitates deep sleep's function of restoring the body. In contrast, during REM sleep much more blood goes to the brain, to facilitate the heightened brain activity of REM dreams.

About 80 percent of people awakened during REM sleep report vivid dreams. As mentioned earlier, dreamlike experiences can occur during stage 1, the transition from wakefulness to sleep. Dreams also occur occasionally during other stages of non-REM sleep. About 5 percent of people awakened during non-REM sleep report dreams. But non-REM dreams are fragmented and inarticulate compared with REM dreams, and they contain fewer identifiable characters and actions. Non-REM dreams are remembered much less vividly than REM dreams.

SLEEP CYCLES

After the first REM period, the sleeper begins the cycle again. Once more, sleep progresses down through stages 2, 3, and 4, followed by the second REM period. The period from sleep onset to the end of the first REM period is called the first *sleep cycle.*

We go through four to six cycles each night, depending on how long we sleep. Each sleep cycle lasts approximately ninety minutes. During the transition among the different sleep stages, our entire physiology alters. This includes such functions as heart rate, respiration, and muscle tone.

Often we awaken after completing a sleep cycle. Usually we fall immediately back to sleep, and we later forget that we awakened. However, sometimes we have difficulty returning to sleep again, as we will see in Chapter 2.

Sleep cycles become increasingly shallower as the night progresses. By the third sleep cycle stage 4 usually disappears, and by the fourth cycle stage 3 usually drops out as well. During the last part of the night, sleep cycles consist of sequences alternating between REM and stage 2, with no deeper sleep. (Stage 1 occurs only when the sleeper awakens during the night. It then serves again as a transition from wakefulness to the deeper sleep stages.)

Most of the restorative effects of a night's sleep come during the first three to five hours, because during that time most deep sleep occurs. Therefore, you can function effectively — if not optimally — after just a few hours of sleep.

Poor sleepers of all ages get more shallow sleep and less deep sleep compared with good sleepers. This problem can be alleviated readily, as you will see in Part IV.

HOW SLEEP CHANGES AS YOU GROW OLDER

Most people begin sleeping less after they enter middle age. Average adult sleep length declines from seven and a half hours in early adulthood to six hours by the seventies.

With increasing age people get less of the deep, restorative sleep of stages 3 and 4, and they awaken more easily during the night. In Figure 1 (page 35) you can see this progression by comparing the sleep of children, young adults, and older adults.

These normal developments of aging need not cause you distress. Chapter 5 explains more about these changes and how to cope with them.

WHY SOME PEOPLE SLEEP BETTER THAN OTHERS

Some people almost always fall asleep easily and sleep soundly through the night. Others have difficulty falling and staying asleep nearly every night. Most of us experience sleep quality somewhere between these two extremes.

Our genetic endowment — what we are born with — plays a large role in determining how well each of us sleeps. In other words, people are born with a tendency toward being good sleepers or poor sleepers. This fact will come as no surprise to parents of more than one child, who often observe that from birth their children have different sleep patterns; siblings may differ greatly in how much sleep they need, how easily they fall asleep, how soundly they sleep through the night, and whether they are "morning people" or "night people."

Research has established the genetic basis of individual differences in sleep patterns. This research includes studies in which identical twins, who have identical sets of genes, show sleep patterns much more similar than the sleep patterns of nonidentical twins, who share fewer genes.

Because of the wide individual differences in sleep quality, you cannot determine how well you sleep by comparing yourself with someone else or with an average. You can judge the quality of your sleep only by comparing how well you sleep now with how well you have usually slept in the past. You should be concerned about your sleep only if it begins to show a significant change from its former pattern. But remember that it is a natural developmental change to sleep less soundly as you grow older.

A genetic basis for the quality of our sleep does not mean that we should be fatalistic about insomnia. Although the pattern and quality of our sleep are determined in part by genetic factors, learned sleep-related habits greatly affect the quality of our sleep. Those of us endowed with a tendency toward poor sleep must be more careful than others about these habits. The chapters of Part IV show how.

2

Insomnia and Other Sleep Problems

SLEEP PROBLEMS CAN BE DIVIDED INTO TWO BASIC CATEGO-
ries: The first is insomnia; the second comprises all other
sleep disorders. This chapter examines both categories.
First, though, let's see how many people have trouble
sleeping.

PREVALENCE OF SLEEP PROBLEMS

Few people are immune from sleep problems. In one
Gallup poll, only 5 percent of adults said that they never
have trouble sleeping. In contrast, about half of adults surveyed report that they have experienced significant sleep
problems at some time in their life.

When people are asked about their *recent* sleep experiences, during the previous year, the figures remain
high. Between 30 and 35 percent — or sixty million American adults — say that they have had some trouble
sleeping during the previous year. And about half of this

group characterize their sleep problems as severe or constant.

Large-scale American surveys regarding sleep problems have produced remarkably consistent results. Sleep problems occur with about the same frequency in urban and rural areas. European sleep surveys report a similar prevalence of sleeplessness.

Sleep problems cause ten million Americans to consult their physicians annually. Despite the fact that sleeping pills can be dangerous and often make a sleep problem worse, twenty-one million prescriptions for sleeping pills are written each year.

In a survey of American households the Nielsen company found that about twenty million people are consistently up watching television between midnight and 3:00 A.M. Many of these people would prefer to be lost in their own dreams, not those of the entertainment industry, but they are kept awake by sleep problems.

Sleep problems are about twice as common among women as men. They are also more prevalent among adults who sleep alone than they are among those who have bed partners. However, most of the people who sleep alone probably sleep worse because they *live* alone, not because they sleep alone. Living alone is often associated with poorer social and emotional adjustment, and increased insomnia is likely to be one manifestation of this poorer adjustment. In fact, we will see in Chapter 13 that couples who are used to sleeping together in a double bed may actually sleep better in separate beds. One person's movements in bed can disturb the bed partner, causing his or her sleep to become shallower.

There is a strong relationship between sleep problems and age. The older we are, the more difficulty we have with sleep. We will explore this phenomenon and what to do about it in Chapter 5.

Now that we have reviewed the prevalence of sleep problems, it is time to examine the two major categories in which sleep problems occur: insomnia and other sleep disorders.

INSOMNIA

On a personal level you know what insomnia is. You may be exhausted from missing sleep the previous night, but you still feel wired as you lie there in bed. Your mind is racing, your muscles are tight, and the more you try to relax, the tenser you become.

Maybe you're worried about a conversation you had during the day, or maybe you're anxious about a meeting at work tomorrow morning. When you count sheep or try to stop thinking, your mind begins to race even faster. Even though you're way behind in your sleep, you can't seem to unwind, let alone drift off.

It might be 11:00 P.M., shortly after you have turned off the light. Or it may be 2:00 A.M., when you awaken after sleeping a couple of hours and can't get back to sleep. Or it's 4:00 A.M., and you know you'll be awake until your alarm clock goes off. Whichever time of the night it is, you find yourself staring at the clock, wondering why you can't sleep again.

As you lie there, you know what the next day will be like. You'll drag through the morning, keeping yourself awake with coffee. In the afternoon you'll grow irritable and have a hard time concentrating. At home that evening, you won't have the energy to do more than watch TV. You'll begin to feel apprehensive as bedtime approaches, because you'll be thinking of the hours you've spent tossing and turning. You'll dread going to bed. And when you turn out the light and lie down, you won't be able to sleep. The cycle will begin again.

Insomnia is real, and it's no fun.

TROUBLE FALLING ASLEEP OR STAYING ASLEEP

The term "insomnia" is actually a misnomer, because it implies a complete lack of sleep. Sleep professionals sometimes refer to insomnia as DIMS, an acronym for "disorders of initiating and maintaining sleep." This term recognizes that insomnia comes in two major types. Some people have difficulty *falling* asleep, and some have difficulty *staying* asleep through the night. Others experience both problems. Still others find that their insomnia shifts over time from a problem with falling asleep to a problem with staying asleep.

One recent survey of more than three thousand adults from age eighteen to seventy-nine asked those people most distressed about their sleep problems when in the night they experienced trouble. Of the group, 37 percent reported difficulty falling asleep, 27 percent reported difficulty staying asleep, and 36 percent were bothered by both problems.

Difficulty falling asleep is the more common type of insomnia among people under forty or fifty. Difficulty staying asleep becomes more common after that age. This condition was aptly described by the writer Franz Kafka: "I fall asleep soundly, but after an hour I wake up, as though I had laid my head in the wrong hole. I . . . have before me anew the labor of falling asleep and I feel myself rejected by sleep."

People with this problem sometimes succeed in falling back asleep. Sometimes they awaken unrefreshed in the predawn hours, unable to fall back to sleep at all. These episodes of insomnia are called early-morning awakening. As we will see in Chapter 9, early-morning awakening occurs often to people suffering from depression.

Even if a person has trouble falling asleep or staying asleep, the problem constitutes significant insomnia only if it interferes with daytime mood or functioning. The seriousness of insomnia is measured not by how little a person sleeps but by how well the person feels and functions the next day.

INSOMNIA SUFFERERS' PERCEPTIONS OF HOW WELL
THEY SLEEP

Despite our genuine distress during bad nights, it can be useful to consider the accuracy of our perception of how well we sleep. People with insomnia tend to overestimate how long it takes them to fall asleep and to underestimate how long they sleep.

One study at Stanford University observed a group of self-reported insomniacs overnight in the sleep laboratory. The next morning, these subjects estimated on average that it had taken them about an hour to fall asleep and that they had slept only four and a half hours. However, recordings of their sleep showed that the subjects had slept much better than they reported. In fact, the subjects on average had taken about fifteen minutes to fall asleep and had slept for six and a half hours.

Sleep recordings show that when chronic insomnia sufferers first fall asleep, they frequently alternate among stage 1, stage 2, and wakefulness. Severe insomniacs usually report that they were still awake if they are aroused from stage 1 — and sometimes from the early part of stage 2. They appear to perceive the onset of sleep at a later time than other people, and they don't perceive themselves as asleep until they are well into stage 2.

Some people go to sleep disorders centers because they believe that they sleep poorly, only to find that objective physiological monitoring shows they sleep much better than they think. Sometimes this insight itself is sufficient to help them stop worrying about their sleep. Clinicians at sleep disorders centers often report this therapeutic effect.

In rare cases people who complain of insomnia actually sleep well, but during the night they dream that they are awake and trying to sleep. Even though they may get a full night of sleep, they awaken in the morning feeling exhausted.

These findings — that insomnia sufferers sometimes sleep better than they think they do — are not intended to minimize the reality and the distress of insomnia. These are facts revealed by research and by the observations of sleep clinicians. It can be useful to know that in some instances, especially when we feel anxious about losing sleep, we may overestimate the amount of sleep loss.

RACING MIND OR TENSE BODY?

In one study, nearly three hundred insomnia sufferers were asked which of two factors seemed to keep them awake as they lay sleepless in bed. The first factor was described as physical arousal at bedtime: feeling restless, sweating, tossing and turning. The second factor was described as mental arousal at bedtime: ruminating, planning, worrying, and difficulty controlling thoughts.

Only 5 percent of these insomnia sufferers said that physical arousal alone described their condition in bed. In contrast, 55 percent said they experienced mental but not physical arousal. Another 35 percent said they experienced both kinds of arousal, and 5 percent said that neither kind of arousal described their insomnia.

Mental arousal, then, is cited more often than physical arousal when people describe their insomnia. That is, even though the body is relaxed, the mind may be racing. Chapter 15 will review in detail several different strategies for coping with physical and mental arousal.

CHILDHOOD-ONSET INSOMNIA

A relatively small number of people begin to suffer during childhood from chronic and relentless insomnia, including both difficulty falling asleep and staying asleep.

The earlier in life a case begins, the more severe it tends to be. Unfortunately, childhood-onset insomnia usually starts at birth and lasts a lifetime.

Childhood-onset insomnia appears to be caused by defects in the neurological system that regulates wakefulness and sleep. Many people with childhood-onset insomnia showed signs of hyperactivity or learning disabilities as children. As adults they may show unusual patterns of brain activity suggestive of neurological impairment.

In the 1982 classic physicians' guide *The Sleep Disorders* (Kalamazoo, Mich.: The Upjohn Company, 1982), psychologist Peter Hauri, director of the Mayo Clinic Sleep Disorders Center, presented a typical case history of childhood-onset insomnia: "Miss E, a 29-year-old secretary, had been an insomniac since birth. In fact, her hospital chart bore a note from the newborn nursery commenting on her remarkable alertness. Miss E's earliest memories were of preschool nights spent sitting quietly by her window for hours, watching the deserted streets below, while her parents slept."

Hauri reported that Miss E was treated successfully with a low dose of the antidepressant Elavil. She has remained on the medication, and her sleep has maintained marked improvement. Every year she withdraws from the medication on a trial basis for a few weeks, only to experience the return of her severe insomnia.

Even though people with childhood-onset insomnia may not be depressed, they sometimes respond well to a low dose of antidepressant drugs. The exact therapeutic action of the drug on sleep is unknown. Other medications have also proved effective with this disorder.

As in all cases of insomnia, medication is not the sole answer. People with childhood-onset insomnia can benefit if they work hard to learn and use the techniques proved to improve sleep for *all* people. Part IV presents these techniques in detail.

CAUSES OF INSOMNIA

Insomnia can be caused by many different factors. Part III describes these causes in detail, but it is useful now — before you begin to diagnose your sleep problem — to survey these factors briefly. That way you will have a better idea of what to look for when you go through the sleep questionnaire and fill out your sleep log.

Sleep Changes with Aging (Chapter 5)

The quality of our sleep changes significantly over the course of a lifetime. Beginning gradually in our thirties and accelerating in our forties and fifties, we sleep less soundly than we used to. In particular, with increasing age many of us experience nighttime awakenings and a subsequent inability to get back to sleep.

We can't reverse these changes and sleep the way we did as children. But it can be comforting just to know that the change in your sleep with age is a normal human development, rather than a sign that there is something wrong with you.

Chapter 5 details how changes in your sleep occur with the aging process. You will also learn how best to cope with these changes.

Medical Conditions and Medication Effects (Chapter 6)

Many physical conditions can disrupt your sleep. It will be obvious to you how some conditions contribute to insomnia. For example, few people sleep well when they have headaches or arthritis pains. But some medical conditions can interfere with sleep in ways that you would not suspect.

Sleep apnea is a syndrome in which breathing ceases for a short time during sleep. The sleeper wakes gasping for breath. This cycle may repeat itself hundreds of times a night. Men over forty with a tendency toward obesity are more likely to have this disorder than are women and younger, thinner men. Snoring is one symptom of sleep apnea, although not all people who snore have apnea.

Some people with sleep apnea report a problem with frequent nighttime awakenings. Others fall asleep quickly after each apnea episode, unaware that they have awakened at all. In the latter case the major complaint is excessive daytime sleepiness — the result of the constant disruption of sleep by the breathing problem.

Restless legs syndrome causes the person to experience strange and unpleasant crawling movements when lying down. Usually this disorder leads to complaints of difficulty falling asleep. A related syndrome, *periodic limb movements,* causes the legs or arms to twitch and jerk during sleep. Often the sleeper is unaware that there is any problem. Because this condition can disrupt sleep without the person's awareness, periodic limb movements often lead to complaints of daytime sleepiness.

Chapter 6 details what to do about these and other physical conditions that can interfere with sleep.

Sleeping Pills (Chapter 7)

Prescription and over-the-counter sleep medications typically lose effectiveness if taken regularly for about a month or longer. They can make your body rely on pills to fall asleep and stay asleep. Then, when you try to sleep without the medication, your insomnia will be much worse than it was originally. For this reason many people become addicted to sleeping pills; they take the pills even though they aren't as effective as they once were, just to avoid the much worse insomnia that results when they try to sleep without medication.

Despite these problems, there are situations in which

sleeping pills are effective and safe. Chapter 7 offers specific guidelines for determining how and when the use of medication is appropriate to help you sleep.

Alcohol, Tobacco, and Caffeine (Chapter 8)

A drink of alcohol within two hours of bedtime may well help you fall asleep initially. But it will very likely cause you to awaken during the night, unable to fall back to sleep.

The nicotine in tobacco is a stimulant, just as caffeine is. Smokers have difficulty falling asleep because of nicotine's stimulating effect. They also tend to awaken during the night because of the withdrawal effects from not taking in nicotine.

The effects of caffeine on sleep vary enormously from person to person. Some people can drink coffee near bedtime and sleep well. Others sleep poorly at night when they eat a chocolate bar in the afternoon. For most people, drinking more than three cups of coffee or cola during the day will interfere with sleep.

Chapter 8 details how these three drugs can interfere with sleep. It also offers suggestions for limiting their sleep-disturbing effects.

Depression (Chapter 9)

Some people feel sad much of the time. They may feel useless or uninterested in people and events around them. Those suffering from depression often experience early-morning awakening. Self-help or professional treatment of depression reduces insomnia in most cases.

Chapter 9 includes a questionnaire to help you determine whether and to what extent you experience depression. It also gives guidelines for self-help treatments, as well as when and how to seek professional help.

Stress and Anxiety (Chapter 10)

Most of us have experienced trouble sleeping because of the everyday stresses of life. It is natural for poor sleep to occur the night after a particularly trying day or the night before an important event. In addition, several anxiety conditions can interfere with sleep. This chapter presents effective techniques that can help you reduce the impact of stress and anxiety on your sleep — and on the rest of your life.

Sleep-Wake Rhythms and Sunday-Night Insomnia (Chapter 11)

Some people can sleep well, but not at the time when they want to. They may sleep fine when they can go to bed late and sleep in late — on weekends or vacations — but not at other times.

Going to bed and getting up at irregular times prevents your body from staying in a natural sleep-wake rhythm. Sometimes daytime naps destabilize our sleep-wake rhythms — particularly when we nap to make up for lost sleep.

Many people sleep exceptionally well on Friday and Saturday nights and then regularly experience insomnia on Sunday nights. This pattern is another sign of a disorder in the body's natural sleep-wake rhythms. Chapter 11 describes ways to cure problems with sleep-wake rhythms.

Conditioned Insomnia (Chapter 12)

Nearly all of us have occasional nights when we don't sleep well. These tend to occur when we are experiencing a particularly stressful time. If the situational stress goes away or diminishes after a few days, as often happens, our insomnia usually disappears as well.

Sometimes, however, the stress lasts for a few weeks or longer. Not surprisingly, the insomnia tends to stay, too. In this situation, there is a danger that the person will learn to associate the sleep environment — the bed and bedroom — with frustrated wakefulness rather than with sleep. Then the insomnia will take on a life of its own, persisting even after the situational stress has gone away.

This disorder is called *conditioned insomnia*. It can be treated with self-help techniques, as you will see in Chapter 12.

OTHER SLEEP DISORDERS

Although insomnia is the most common sleep disorder, it is not the only one. This section examines sleep disorders other than insomnia. Because these disorders are sometimes related to insomnia, it can be helpful to review them briefly.

NIGHTMARES

Chapter 1 showed that dreams occur about every ninety minutes, during REM sleep. Nightmares are long dreams that can last twenty minutes or longer; they tend to occur late in the night, when the sleeper experiences the longest periods of REM. Nightmares cause anxiety intense enough to awaken the sleeper. Often the person can recall the dream in detail.

About 5 percent of adults experience current problems with nightmares. Another 5 percent have had difficulty with them in the past.

Nightmares involve themes of intense fear, danger, being chased, or a feeling of being overwhelmed. They are a normal part of the human experience. The average adult is likely to have at least one nightmare a year. Some people are more susceptible to nightmares than others. Women report more nightmares than men do.

Nightmares are sometimes triggered by a trauma in the person's history. Accident victims and combat veterans often report nightmares that are related to traumatizing events they have experienced. In most cases, the frequency and severity of the nightmares lessen with the passage of time.

Certain people experience nightmares during *REM rebound*. This condition occurs when a person has been taking a drug — such as an antidepressant or marijuana — that suppresses REM sleep. After the person stops taking the drug, REM and associated dreaming increase to a level higher than they originally were, as if to make up for the dream time lost when the person was taking REM-suppressing medication. If the person has been deprived of REM for a long period, subsequent dreams during REM rebound can take on a nightmarish quality.

Some people cope with nightmare-inspired anxieties by writing down the contents of the nightmares in dream journals. They believe that the process of recording and reviewing their dreams helps them gain insight — on their own or with a psychotherapist — into events or unresolved emotional concerns that may have contributed to the nightmares. If you choose to keep a dream journal, it is important to write down the dream immediately, before it fades from memory.

Other people view nightmares simply as frightening inconveniences with no real significance. They cope with them by forgetting them and returning to sleep. If they are too upset to sleep immediately, they redirect their attention with reading or some other distracting activity until they can fall asleep again. You are the one who can best decide which of these two approaches makes more sense for you.

NIGHT TERRORS

As we have seen, a nightmare is a frightful dream that happens during REM sleep. People typically describe anything that causes fear or anxiety during sleep as a nightmare. But a different phenomenon sometimes occurs.

In contrast to nightmares, which often are recalled as a sequence of events, *night terrors* — sometimes called *sleep terrors* — usually leave people unable to describe anything other than a feeling of intense fear and panic. Those who can recall something usually describe a single image that is terrifying and overpowering.

A night terror begins when the person suddenly sits up in bed with a wide-eyed stare, the face contorted. The person may kick and thrash about in bed, flailing the arms as the body fights an unknown dread danger. The person often screams and may even run around the room. This is very different from someone having a nightmare, whose body, except for the eyes, remains immobilized during the experience.

A person in a night terror trembles, sweats, and shows a rapid increase in heart rate. If you try to talk to someone having a night terror, the person usually will not respond. Because the person is not really awake, he or she does not know you are there.

Don't try to wake someone in the grip of a night terror because he or she will become confused and frightened at your presence. Usually the person falls back asleep before long and recalls nothing about the experience the next morning.

Night terrors occur during the deepest sleep of the night, the delta sleep of stages 3 and 4. Because most deep sleep comes early in the night, a night terror almost always occurs during the first half of the night's sleep; most occur during the first sleep cycle, within sixty to ninety minutes after falling asleep.

Chapter 1 showed that it is very difficult to wake a person from deep delta sleep. Some people cannot fully awaken at all when they are sleeping deeply. If something disturbs them while they are in delta sleep, the brain functions as if it is half asleep and half awake. This confused condition is the setting for a night terror.

Night terrors are more apt to occur during particularly stressful times. Because they occur during deep sleep, and because children have more deep sleep than adults, they are more likely to experience night terrors. Two to 3 percent of children have night terrors. Usually the problem disappears by adolescence. However, night terrors can persist into adulthood, and in rare instances they first arise in adulthood.

Children or adults susceptible to night terrors can reduce their frequency by decreasing the amount of deep sleep they get. It may sound paradoxical, but the way to decrease your deep sleep is by *sleeping longer* because the longer you sleep, the less deeply you sleep.

As we will see in Chapter 16, an important step in overcoming insomnia is to do the opposite: sleep *less*, so that you fall asleep more quickly and your sleep becomes deeper.

SLEEPWALKING

Three to 4 percent of adults sleepwalk at least once. In the past, it was thought that sleepwalkers were acting out their dreams. Now it is known that sleepwalking begins during deep sleep, rather than the dream time of REM. Like night terrors, sleepwalking — or *somnambulism* — is caused by incomplete arousal from deep sleep. In fact, the same people are prone to sleepwalking and to night terrors. Extreme sleep deprivation can lead to either disorder when the person sleeps again, because sleep deprivation is followed by an increase in deep sleep. Research suggests that a genetic component contributes to both these disorders.

The brain of a sleepwalker is partly asleep and partly awake. Some kind of sensory mechanism appears to operate, because a sleepwalking person usually avoids obstacles, although he or she may also trip over a chair or fall down a stairway. Sometimes the sleepwalker can perform a task such as opening a door, filling a glass from the faucet, or even starting up a car. However, there is no logic in the sleepwalker's behavior; the person may open a closet door and walk inside, fill a glass of water but leave it on the counter, or start a car without driving anywhere.

The sleepwalker's eyes stare from an expressionless face. He or she usually does not respond to other people's attempts to converse. Sleepwalking episodes typically last less than ten minutes.

In most cases, a sleepwalker remembers nothing about the episode the next day. Don't wake a sleepwalker, because he or she may become disoriented and frightened to be out of bed at night. Just stand by and be prepared to help if the person approaches a dangerous situation. Usually a sleepwalker returns to bed on his or her own after the episode has run its course. Sometimes a sleepwalker can be guided gently back to bed.

Because of the dangers of physical injury, it is best to take some basic precautions in a home with a sleepwalking person. Try to have the sleepwalker sleep on the first floor. Block stairways, lock outside doors, put away dangerous objects, and hide the car keys.

SLEEP TALKING

You may recall that during REM sleep the body's large muscles are semiparalyzed. Occasionally, though, the sleeper is able to use speech muscles during REM. In these instances the person sometimes verbalizes what he or she is dreaming about.

Occasionally people in REM can hear and understand

what someone else says to them. They can incorporate this talk into their dreams and respond to it verbally.

Sleep talking also can occur during stages 1 and 2 and — as with night terrors and sleepwalking — during partial arousal from deep sleep. Sleep talking during deep sleep consists of incomprehensible mumbles, in contrast with the relatively clear talking during REM sleep.

People rarely recall talking in their sleep, even if wakened right after the episode.

SNORING

We learned in the earlier discussion of sleep apnea that snoring is a symptom of that disorder. That is, all apnea sufferers snore. However, the reverse is *not* true. Not all people who snore have sleep apnea.

About half of all adults snore from time to time, and one-fourth snore regularly. In a Gallup poll, 7 percent of men and 18 percent of women reported that their bed partners' snoring disturbed their sleep. Snoring increases in frequency with age. Until late adulthood, many more men snore than women. Among people between thirty and thirty-five, about 20 percent of men snore, compared with just 5 percent of women. But by age sixty, fully 40 percent of women snore, compared with 60 percent of men at that age.

More than three hundred devices to reduce snoring have been patented. They include mouth gags, muzzles, and electrical currents that shock a sleeper when snoring begins. These devices are rarely effective, but here are some self-help measures that do prevent or reduce snoring for many people:

- *Sleep with more than one pillow, to keep your head elevated.*

- *Sleep on your side rather than on your back. One way to stay off your back is to place a tennis ball or other small object in a sock and pin the sock onto the back of your nightclothes.*

- *Use a humidifier in your bedroom, because moist air reduces snoring.*

- *Avoid smoking and drinking, either of which can cause or worsen snoring.*

- *Lose excess weight, which contributes to snoring.*

In extreme cases, surgery can reduce the severity of a snoring problem by increasing airflow in the airway.

NIGHT SWEATS

Heavy sweating at night often occurs in women during menopause. Profuse and persistent perspiring at night can also be a symptom of serious physical disease, such as tuberculosis or a thyroid infection. If you sweat at night but don't have a fever, you need to discuss the symptom with your physician.

EXCESSIVE DAYTIME SLEEPINESS

Between 1 and 4 percent of people have trouble staying awake during the day. If you often fall asleep when you don't intend to, you may not be getting enough sleep at night: You might simply be going to bed too late or getting up too early, or you might be a long sleeper who needs up to ten hours of nightly sleep. Try scheduling one or two hours' more sleep each night, and see if this reduces your daytime sleepiness.

However, if sleeping longer at night doesn't help, you may need to be evaluated at a sleep disorders center (Appendix 6). Although excessive daytime sleepiness is much rarer as a chief complaint than insomnia, people with this problem constitute about half of all patients evaluated at sleep disorders centers. Excessive daytime sleepiness is a symptom of several medical sleep disorders, and a sleep evaluation is often necessary to diagnose the problem.

Earlier in this chapter we saw that people with sleep apnea and periodic limb movements often are unaware that they have a medical problem. Their major complaint is excessive daytime sleepiness, because they don't even realize their nighttime sleep is being disrupted.

Several other factors can also cause extreme daytime sleepiness.

Narcolepsy

This is a syndrome in which a person experiences attacks of daytime sleepiness that are sudden and overwhelming. These attacks can last from a few seconds up to an hour or more; on average, they last about two minutes.

The syndrome is also characterized by *cataplexy*, a loss of muscle tone triggered by strong emotions, such as anger, fear, and excitement, including laughter. Because of the loss of muscle tone, cataplexy can cause the person to become weak in the knees or slump to the ground.

Some narcoleptics exhibit periods of *automatic behavior*, during which they behave normally, but after which they are unable to recall anything they have done. For example, a person with narcolepsy may drive fifty miles past the right exit when commuting home on an interstate highway.

Although narcoleptics may sleep eight hours or more a night, many feel drowsy all day. Paradoxically, they often report nighttime insomnia. Some narcoleptics don't realize they have the disorder; they think that their attacks of daytime sleepiness are simply a consequence of insomnia.

Between two and five people in a thousand suffer from narcolepsy. The disorder is genetically transmitted. It occurs with equal frequency in males and females. Usually it appears between early adolescence and age thirty, and it lasts the rest of the person's life. At present there is no cure, but stimulant medications — sometimes in combination with antidepressants — can reduce its severity.

Taking brief naps (fifteen to thirty minutes) in the morning and afternoon can help avert narcolepsy episodes. Getting plenty of sleep at night —enough to awaken spontaneously in the morning without an alarm clock — also minimizes the problem for some narcoleptics.

Kleine-Levin Syndrome

This rare disorder is another cause of excessive daytime sleepiness. It is characterized by periods of extreme sleepiness that alternate with periods of normal sleep behavior. The Kleine-Levin syndrome primarily affects teenage males.

During sleepy phases, the person can sleep as long as twenty-two hours a day. Someone with this disorder often exhibits a voracious appetite and displays sexual exhibitionism toward members of both sexes. Severe irritability or confusion may also be present. Drug treatment with lithium carbonate can reduce the severity of the Kleine-Levin syndrome. The disorder usually disappears spontaneously before the age of forty.

Menstrual-Related Sleepiness

This phenomenon is experienced by many women. Because estrogen and progesterone influence sleep, most women report that their sleep is better or worse at different times of their menstrual cycles. For some women, excessive sleepiness is associated with menstrual periods or premenstrual syndrome.

Extreme sleepiness can also be an early sign of pregnancy. During pregnancy women often sleep as much as two hours more than their usual average.

Other Medical Syndromes

Hypothyroidism, hypoglycemia, and diabetes sometimes cause excessive sleepiness. Chapter 6 examines the effects of medical disorders on sleep.

REM SLEEP BEHAVIOR DISORDER

In Chapter 1 we saw that during REM periods our brain commands the body's muscles to act out the events in the dream. For example, if we dream about walking, our brain tells the leg muscles to walk. However, a mechanism in our brainstem paralyzes all the body's muscles — except for our eyes — during REM. This prevents us from carrying out the brain's orders.

In rare instances sleepers *do* act out their dreams. This condition was first identified in 1983 at the Minnesota Regional Sleep Disorders Center. In that case, a sixty-seven-year-old man gashed his forehead when he ran into his bedroom dresser while dreaming that he was a football player.

The condition in which sleepers act out their dreams is known as *REM sleep behavior disorder.* It is most likely to affect men over fifty. About 85 percent of people with REM sleep behavior disorder injure themselves during an episode, and nearly half injure their bed partners. In most cases, the sedative clonazepam suppresses the symptoms of this dangerous sleep disorder.

Part II
Let's Diagnose Your Sleep Problem

CONSIDER THESE THREE FACTS:

- *Although there are similarities among sleep problems, each person's sleep problem is unique.*
- *Each person's sleep problem has a particular cause or set of causes.*
- *Sleep problems with different causes require different solutions.*

For these reasons, the most effective way to begin solving your sleep problem is to *diagnose* it, or determine its cause.

The two chapters in Part II provide tools for diagnosing your particular sleep problem. Chapter 3 presents a diagnostic questionnaire designed to help you find out what causes your sleepless nights. Your responses will help you identify and understand some of the contributing factors.

Then you can focus on the sections of this book that address those factors.

In going through the questionnaire, you may recognize one or two factors that appear to be obvious contributors to your particular sleep problem. For example, you may find that the cause of your sleep problem is a nightcap and that the solution is as simple as having your evening drink with dinner instead. Or you may find that several factors contribute to your sleeplessness, and therefore the solution will involve several steps. Nearly all readers who complete the sleep questionnaire will recognize items that help them diagnose their sleep problem.

Chapter 4 presents the second diagnostic tool — an optional sleep log, in which you record how well you sleep each night, as well as certain aspects of your behavior that day. Completing a sleep log for one or two weeks will enable you to test the accuracy of your hypotheses about the cause or causes of your sleep problem.

Completing the questionnaire and sleep log will enable most readers to diagnose their case of insomnia. But don't worry if you don't succeed in diagnosing yours; not all people can successfully observe and monitor their behavior, and not all are willing to keep a sleep log. Regardless of the cause of your insomnia, if you follow the steps in Part IV, you will improve the quality of your sleep.

3

A Diagnostic Sleep Questionnaire

THIS CHAPTER WILL HELP YOU COME UP WITH EDUCATED guesses — or hypotheses — about the cause or causes of your sleep problem. Go through all twenty-six items of the questionnaire. As you answer the questions, you may want to make notes in the margin or on a piece of paper. Your answers and the explanations with each question will show you where in the book to focus your efforts at solving your sleep problem.

Going through the questionnaire will help you generate hypotheses about what may cause your insomnia. The next step is to test each hypothesis, to determine whether or not a given factor does in fact interfere with your sleep. You will do this by keeping a sleep log, which is explained in the next chapter. Testing your hypotheses is an optional step, but a very useful one if you are willing to monitor your behavior with a sleep log for a week or two.

1. *When you lose sleep at night, do you feel tired or drowsy the next day? Does this drowsiness interfere with your work or your social life?*

These two related questions will help determine whether you really have insomnia. If you sleep little at night but feel rested during the day, review the material in Chapter 1 regarding short sleepers and long sleepers. One in five adults is simply a short sleeper, needing less than six hours a night. Often a short sleeper worries about not getting enough sleep — particularly if his or her bed partner sleeps longer.

As long as you feel reasonably rested and alert during the daytime, don't worry if you don't sleep a lot. It's likely that you are a short sleeper. Just enjoy the extra time you have each night, and use it to relax or to get things done.

2. *How many times do you awaken during the night? Is it difficult for you to get back to sleep?*

Most good sleepers actually wake for just a few seconds at least five times each night. However, they quickly fall back asleep and in the morning forget that they have awakened. Awakening is not a problem in itself, but being unable to get back to sleep is a problem.

Nighttime awakenings become more frequent as we grow older. Chapter 5 shows how to cope with this normal development.

The physiological effects of alcohol or tobacco can cause nighttime awakenings. If this might be the case with you, look at the material in Chapter 8.

In Chapter 15, you will learn ways to put yourself back to sleep after waking at night. You also will see what to do if you can't get back to sleep.

3. *Do you often awaken in the predawn hours to find yourself unable to return to sleep at all?*

If you wake too early in the morning, you may be going to bed too early in the evening, and your current sleep schedule may have more hours scheduled for sleep than you actually need. To find out if this is the case with you, for a week go to sleep an hour or two later in the evening. If you wake up closer to the hour you want, you may have been trying to sleep too long.

Some older adults habitually go to bed early in the evening and consequently waken long before dawn. Chapter 5 shows ways to prevent this problem.

Awakening early in the morning and being unable to return to sleep also can be a sign of depression. See the discussion in Chapter 9 if you suspect this may be the case.

4. *Are you under a physician's care for any medical condition?*

   Many kinds of body disorders can disrupt sleep. If you have an acute or chronic medical condition, read Chapter 6.

5. *Do you snore, or do you suspect you might have problems breathing while lying down?*

   Chapter 2 presents ways to reduce a snoring problem. But snoring sometimes signals a more serious sleep disorder. If you snore or suspect that you may have breathing problems during sleep, look carefully at the discussion of sleep apnea in Chapter 6.

6. *While lying down, do you ever experience unpleasant sensations in your legs? Do your legs sometimes kick or jerk in bed? Or do you awaken with your lower leg muscles feeling uncomfortable or with your bedding severely disarrayed?*

   As many as 5 to 10 percent of adults have involuntary leg movements that wake them at night. If you recognize any of the above indications, read about periodic limb movements and restless leg syndrome in Chapter 6.

7. *Do you have a fairly regular bedtime and wake-up time? Or do you go to bed and get up at very different times from day to day?*

   A regular sleep-wake schedule helps induce sleepiness at bedtime. If your bedtime and wake-up time are irregular, you will benefit from reading the information in Chapters 11 and 14.

8. *Is it harder to fall asleep on Sunday night than on other nights? Do you feel more tired on Monday morning than on other days?*

   Sunday-night insomnia is a common problem that is easily remedied, as you will see in Chapter 11.

9. *Are you most alert late in the evening? Do you have difficulty falling asleep until a very late hour and difficulty awakening early in the morning? Do you sleep many hours later on weekends, to make up for sleep you lost during the week?*

   This pattern of behavior is known as *delayed sleep phase syndrome*. It is most common among adolescents and younger adults, and it is estimated to cause about 10 percent of chronic insomnia cases. Chapter 11 explains ways to minimize this syndrome and normalize sleep patterns.

10. *Do you typically feel sleepy in the evening, falling asleep by 8:00 P.M.? Do you awaken by 3:00 or 4:00 A.M., unable to sleep longer?*

    This pattern of behavior is the opposite of delayed sleep phase syndrome discussed above. It occurs most often in old age, and it sometimes is associated with depression.
    If you fall asleep and awaken earlier than you would like, read the section on *advanced sleep phase*

syndrome in Chapter 11. In addition, complete the depression checklist in Chapter 9, to determine if depression contributes to your sleep problem.

11. *After you awaken in the morning, do you usually lie in bed, drifting in and out of sleep?*

It can be pleasant to rest in bed in the morning, and some people can do it with no negative effects. However, most insomnia sufferers will worsen their sleep problems by stretching out the length of time they sleep and rest in bed. This habit tends to make sleep become shallower, as you will see in Chapter 16.

12. *Do you often nap during the day? Do you nap nearly every day or only on those days when you haven't slept well the previous night?*

Some people do well by napping regularly. However, napping can interfere with nighttime sleep. And napping to make up for lost sleep will worsen your insomnia problem. See the information on napping in Chapter 14.

13. *Are you in your forties or older, and do you think you don't sleep as well as you used to?*

Around this age, most people begin to awaken more often during the night and have a harder time getting back to sleep than when they were younger. Simply knowing that this pattern is normal can dispel some worry about sleeplessness. Chapter 5 looks at ways for older adults to sleep better.

14. *Do you ever use prescription drugs or over-the-counter medications to help you sleep?*

Sleeping pills are sometimes effective when used short term for a situational crisis. However, they often compound a sleep problem rather than help it. If you take sleep medication, be sure to read Chapter 7.

15. *If you take sleep medication, are the pills as effective as they once were? Or have you found that the pills don't work as well as they did when you first started taking them?*

Many medications, including all sleep medications, over time lose the effectiveness they initially had. The phenomenon of a drug becoming less effective is known as *tolerance*. Drug tolerance leads to the need for increasingly larger doses to achieve the initial effect achieved with smaller doses. Drug tolerance is one of two hallmarks of physical dependence. The use of sleeping pills is discussed in Chapter 7.

16. *If you often take sleep medication, have you found that you can't sleep on nights when you don't take a sleeping pill?*

The second hallmark of physical drug dependence is *withdrawal*. This term is used to describe any symptom that appears when a drug that is taken regularly is discontinued. When sleeping pills are taken regularly and then stopped, the syndrome that appears is *rebound insomnia,* which causes your sleep to be worse than it was before you started taking sleeping pills. If you may be in this situation, read Chapter 7. Then make an appointment with your physician, to discuss dependence on sleep medication.

17. *Do you take any prescription drugs or over-the-counter medications for conditions other than sleep problems?*

Many medications can cause insomnia. See the information in Chapter 6 regarding the side effects on sleep of different medications.

18. *Do you smoke, drink alcohol, or consume caffeine in any form?*

Any of these three drugs can disrupt sleep severely, particularly when taken during the evening. Alcohol might help you fall asleep more easily, but it is likely to make you awaken during the night. Read Chapter 8 if alcohol, tobacco, or caffeine is part of your life.

19. *Do you get vigorous exercise at least three times a week?*

Regular exercise helps you fall asleep more easily and sleep more deeply. The best time to exercise to promote sleep is in the late afternoon or early evening. Exercise earlier in the day will have a less beneficial effect. And vigorous exercise shortly before bedtime will actually interfere with sleep.

If you aren't exercising regularly, read the sections on exercise in Chapters 9 and 14. You will see how exercise alters body temperature to help you sleep more soundly, and you will learn tips for making exercise work best to improve your sleep.

20. *Do you experience at least mild levels of depression, anxiety, or stress during the day or night?*

In some cases, nighttime insomnia is a reflection of daytime stress, anxiety, or depression. Chapters 9 and 10 contain questionnaires to help you evaluate your emotional state, as well as techniques for improving it.

21. *Do daytime worries keep you awake at night?*

This is a common experience of insomnia sufferers. Chapter 10 surveys ways to help you manage daytime stress and reduce its impact on your sleep. Chapters 14 and 15 show how to leave daytime worries behind you at bedtime.

22. *Do you sleep poorly the night after a particularly stressful day or evening?*

   It is not unusual for insomnia to follow a difficult day. To learn how to reduce this problem, read Chapter 10.

23. *Do you have a hard time sleeping the night before an important event, such as an examination, a job interview, or your child's wedding?*

   This phenomenon is also common. Fortunately, your body's adrenaline helps you function well at a critical event, even if you have slept poorly the night before. Techniques to reduce the problem are presented in Part IV.

24. *Do you usually perform enjoyable, relaxing activities — such as listening to music, reading, or watching TV — in the hours before bedtime? Or do you instead have family arguments or do take-home work from your job?*

   Engaging in stressful activities before bedtime can disrupt your sleep. Chapter 14 shows how to prevent this problem.

25. *Do you sleep better almost anywhere but in your bed? Do you tend to fall asleep unintentionally while reading or watching TV, only to find that you can't sleep when you move to your bed?*

   Some people sleep well on vacation in hotel rooms, but not in their own beds. They fall asleep readily while reading or watching TV in the living room — but again, not in bed. These people have what is known as conditioned insomnia, or learned insomnia. It develops when individuals have lain awake so often in their darkened bedrooms that they have learned to associate the bedroom with frustration, anxiety, and sleeplessness, rather than with sleep.

Conditioned insomnia is a disorder that can be treated successfully, as Chapter 12 shows.

26. *Do you work the night shift or rotating shifts?*

People who work nights or rotate day and night shifts often have sleep problems because they cannot adjust their body's sleep-wake rhythms to the shifts they work. Appendix 3 reviews ways of coping with this problem.

4

An Optional Sleep Log

AFTER YOU COMPLETE THE SLEEP QUESTIONNAIRE IN Chapter 3, you may have some hypotheses about the cause of your insomnia. Or you may be as puzzled as you were to begin with. In either case, a good next step is to fill out the sleep log in this chapter. Do this each morning for a week. In some instances, it is necessary to fill out the log for two weeks.

There are three reasons to keep a sleep log. First, and most important, *the sleep log will help you test your hypotheses about the cause of your insomnia.* That is, by filling out the log, you can determine whether each hypothesis is accurate.

The second reason to complete a sleep log is that *by recording sleep and sleep-related behaviors, you will become more objectively aware of your sleep patterns.* Some people who believe that they typically sleep only a few hours a night find out through their logs that, in fact, they sleep much more. Other people who believe that their insomnia occurs almost every night may discover that it occurs less frequently. This knowledge in itself can be reassuring.

There is a third reason to complete a sleep log: *The very act of monitoring your behavior can help bring about the desired changes.* This principle often is seen in behavioral self-management. For example, smokers usually smoke less during a period when they are completing a log of the cigarettes they smoke. Overeaters tend to eat less when they monitor their food intake.

Monitoring your own sleep behavior encourages you to think about your sleep and the factors that may affect it. Self-monitoring also makes it more likely that you actually will take the intervention steps that you plan. For example, if you plan to get out of bed as soon as you awaken in the morning — a good idea, as Chapter 16 shows — you are more likely to carry through if you know that you will be recording your behavior in the sleep log.

WHAT IF YOU DON'T WANT TO KEEP A LOG?

Many people don't like the idea of keeping a sleep log. This resistance occurs whether people use self-help techniques alone, work with a behavioral therapist, or undergo treatment at a sleep disorders center. Some find it overwhelming to think about keeping track of one more thing, when their daily routines already seem too complicated. Some are uncomfortable with the process of taking a close look at their behavior. However, keeping a sleep log is neither tedious nor time-consuming. Even if you feel uncertain, make a real effort to complete the sleep log, because it will help you diagnose your insomnia.

Fill out the sleep log on page 80 every morning for a week. The information you enter will give you a record of how long and how well you sleep each night. It also will provide a record of the factors that may influence your sleep, such as alcohol or caffeine consumption, daytime or evening stress, exercise, or a disordered sleep schedule. Monitoring this information will be an important step toward improving the quality of your sleep.

However, if in the end you choose not to fill out the sleep log, or if you complete the log but can't detect any patterns to your insomnia, you still can carry on with the program to reduce or eliminate your insomnia. Rely on what you learned from the sleep questionnaire in the previous chapter. Then look at the chapters in Part III. You'll probably recognize factors that contribute to your own insomnia. If you do, you can take steps to change them.

Even if you read Part III and still don't recognize the cause of your problem, Part IV will help. It details a program that helps virtually all insomnia sufferers improve their sleep significantly, regardless of the cause of their particular case of insomnia.

HOW TO SET UP YOUR SLEEP LOG

Look at the sample sleep log on page 80. You need to make at least seven photocopies of this log, one to fill out each morning for at least a week. You might want to have the photocopier enlarge the copies, to make the log easier to write on.

Fill out your sleep log within about thirty minutes after awakening each morning. Just guess the approximate times. What is most important is your overall opinion of how well you slept. As you can see in Figure 4-1, you need to record the following information for the *previous* day and evening:

1. The time you turned out the lights and tried to sleep
2. How difficult it was for you to fall asleep
3. The number of awakenings during the night
4. How long you were awake during each awakening
5. When you last awakened this morning and the total time you slept last night
6. How rested you feel this morning

DAILY SLEEP LOG

Name _____

Last night was (circle one): Su M T W Th F Sat   Last night's date: _____

PART I: LAST NIGHT'S SLEEP QUALITY

1. What time did you turn out the light and try to sleep last night?
   _____

2. How difficult was it for you to fall asleep? (Circle one.)

            1   2   3   4   5

   Not very difficult   Extremely difficult

3. How many times did you awaken during the night? _____

4. Record how many minutes you were awake for each awakening
   you listed above in question 3. _____   _____   _____

5. What is the last time you awakened this morning?_____What is
   the total time you slept last night? _____ hours, _____ minutes.

6. How rested do you feel this morning? (Circle one.)

            1   2   3   4   5

   Very rested   Poorly rested

7. Rate the overall quality of last night's sleep. (Circle one.)

            1   2   3   4   5

   Excellent   Very poor

PART II: BEHAVIOR YESTERDAY AND LAST NIGHT

8. If you napped yesterday: When? _____ For how long? _____

9. For each of the variables you monitered, describe what occurred
   yesterday.   Low   High

Variable 1 (Variable: _____) Rating if appropriate: 1 2 3 4 5
Observation: _____

                                 Low   High
Variable 2 (Variable: _____) Rating if appropriate: 1 2 3 4 5
Observation: _____

                                 Low   High
Variable 3 (Variable: _____) Rating if appropriate: 1 2 3 4 5
Observation: _____

                                 Low   High
Variable 4 (Variable: _____) Rating if appropriate: 1 2 3 4 5
Observation: _____

Figure 4-1

Daily Sleep Log

7. The overall quality of last night's sleep
8. If you napped yesterday, when and for how long
9. Your observations of what occurred yesterday with each of the sleep-related variables you are monitoring

The first seven items will be relatively easy to complete. However, the last item, No. 9, will take some thought on your part. This information may be more difficult to complete, but it is important. In this item you will record the factors that might influence your particular case of insomnia. By completing the questionnaire in Chapter 3, you came up with hypotheses about possible sleep-influencing factors. Because these factors can vary from day to day, they are called *variables*.

There are two parts to your record keeping on item No. 9. First, you need to jot down the variables you are monitoring — for example, exercise, caffeine use, daytime stress, evening worrying. Write down the variables beforehand, so you don't have to try to remember them all when you fill out your sleep log each morning. Second, you need to record what occurred with each of these variables.

MONITOR THE VARIABLES THAT MIGHT INFLUENCE YOUR INSOMNIA

You may be asking yourself what exactly you should record on the log for the variables under item No. 9. There is no simple answer. Each case of insomnia is different, and each person must identify and record the variables that seem to influence his or her own case of insomnia. Clients who consult sleep specialists and even patients who are evaluated at sleep disorders centers are asked to hypothesize possible causes of their sleep problems. The person with the sleep problem best knows what might be causing it.

The best way to identify variables to monitor is by reviewing your responses to the questionnaire in Chapter 3.

If you answer the questions carefully and honestly, you almost certainly will discover at least one possible cause of your sleep problem. Most insomnia sufferers will recognize several factors that may influence how well they sleep at night.

Choose two to four variables that you think may contribute to your insomnia. Limit your monitoring to no more than four variables, because it can be difficult to keep track of more than four simultaneously.

For example, after filling out the questionnaire, you may suspect that four variables might influence how well you sleep that night: tobacco use, afternoon naps, daytime stress, and evening feelings of depression. After you identify these hypotheses, you will record data about each of them in item No. 9 of your sleep log. That is, you record the extent to which each factor occurred on the day just before your night's sleep.

If you are having difficulty coming up with variables that may influence your sleep, examine this list of possible variables. Beneath each variable is a suggestion for how to monitor it from day to day.

1. *Is Sunday night your worst sleep night?*

    Monitor this by comparing the quality of your sleep on Sunday night with other nights during the week.

2. *Is your night's sleep poor after a day on which you have napped?*

    Chart when and for how long you nap. Then compare your night's sleep after you have napped with nights when you haven't napped.

3. *Do you sleep worse when you drink alcohol in the evening?*

    Chart how much and when in the evening you

drink. Then compare how well you sleep after evenings with different amounts of alcohol at different times before you go to bed.

4. *Do you sleep worse when you use tobacco in the evening?*

    Chart when and how much you smoke during the evenings. Then compare how well you sleep after days with different amounts of tobacco.

5. *Do you sleep worse when you take caffeine in any form?*

    Chart when and how much caffeine you ingest. (See Chapter 8 for foods that contain caffeine.) Then compare how well you sleep after days with different amounts of caffeine.

6. *Is your sleep affected by eating close to bedtime?*

    Chart when and how much you eat in the evening. Then compare the quality of your sleep after an evening snack with your sleep on an empty stomach.

7. *Do you sleep worse on days when you don't exercise vigorously?*

    Chart the type, time, and length of each day's exercise. Then compare how well you sleep after days with different types and lengths of exercise. Also compare your night's sleep when you exercise at different times of the day.

8. *Do you sleep worse after a particularly stressful day or evening?*

    Chart stressful events during the day and evening. Rate the day's or evening's stress level on the sleep log's five-point scale. Then compare your sleep after a stressful day or evening with your sleep after a day or evening with little stress.

9. *Do you sleep worse the night before a "big day," when you will give a speech, take an exam, or do some other important activity?*

   Compare your sleep on nights before important events with your sleep on other nights.

10. *Do you sleep better in places other than your bed?*

    Compare your sleep in your own bed with your sleep at other places.

11. *Do you sleep better after you read or watch TV in bed?*

    Compare your sleep on nights after you read or watch TV in bed with your sleep on other nights.

12. *Do you sleep better alone or with your bed partner?*

    Compare your sleep on nights alone with nights when you share the bed.

13. *Do you sleep better on nights after you engage in sex before sleep?*

    Compare your sleep on nights when you have sex at bedtime with your sleep on other nights.

Wherever a variable can be quantified, it is helpful to record the degree to which it occurs. One way to record the degree of a particular variable is to rate it on a scale of one to five. Using a five-point rating scale is a simple way to quantify many variables that differ by degree, particularly such "feeling" variables as anxiety, depression, and happiness. Along with the number, it is good to add a few written observations regarding what occurred and how you felt about it.

CORRELATE YOUR DAY AND EVENING VARIABLES WITH THE
QUALITY OF YOUR NIGHT'S SLEEP

After you have recorded the information on your sleep
log for a week, the next step is to analyze the information.
Here you correlate the quality of your night's sleep with
each of the variables you monitored on your log. The word
"correlate" simply means to determine how two things relate to each other.

This means that you examine nights when you slept relatively well and when you slept relatively poorly, and you
investigate to what extent your two to four variables occurred during the days and evenings preceding those
nights' sleep. This process enables you to test if the variables you monitored do in fact precede — and likely cause
— your insomnia.

Most people with insomnia don't have problems sleeping every night. Even severe insomnia sufferers usually
have one or two nights in a week when they sleep reasonably well. Begin by identifying the one or more nights during the week when you slept relatively well and the one
or more nights when you slept poorly. If you slept poorly
every night, try to identify one night when you slept a little
less poorly than the others. For example, if your log shows
that you typically slept just four or five hours a night but
that on one night you slept six hours, you can define that
as a "good" night's sleep.

The simplest way to identify nights with good and poor
sleep is to examine item No. 7 on the log, in which you
rated the overall quality of each night's sleep. You may
also want to examine item Nos. 2 through 6. *You* are the
one who can best decide what constitutes good and poor
nights of sleep for you. Some people are especially distressed about taking a long time to fall asleep, and others
are more concerned about nighttime awakenings.

After you have identified one or more good nights and one or more poor nights, examine your logs to see what was happening with the variables you monitored during the day before those nights' sleep. For example, you might find that whether or not you experienced evening feelings of depression made no real difference in your sleep that night. But you might find that afternoon naps and evening caffeine use *did* make a difference. That is, you may find that when you nap in the afternoon, you sleep particularly poorly that night. And you may find that you sleep poorly at night when you have had caffeine even eight hours earlier.

A SAMPLE SLEEP LOG

To see how the diagnostic process works, let's look at the completed sample sleep logs on pages 87–88. These were filled out by an attorney in her forties. When Ms. Frazier began the program, she had no idea which factors might be causing good or bad sleep. In fact, she believed that her nights of poor sleep occurred randomly. But despite this skepticism, she went through the questionnaire. After completing it, she thought that sleep might conceivably be affected by four factors: exercise, alcohol use, job-related stress, and having a bedtime snack. She decided to monitor all four variables.

After filling out a sleep log every night for a week, Ms. Frazier analyzed the information by correlating good and bad nights of sleep with the three variables she monitored. Let's see how she did it.

Occasionally Ms. Frazier had difficulty falling asleep. However, she was concerned mainly about awakening during the night and being unable to return to sleep. So when she went night by night through the week's sleep logs, she paid particular attention to item Nos. 3 and 4, which record the number and length of nighttime awakenings.

When she compared this information across the week,

DAILY SLEEP LOG

Name __Judy Frazier__

Last night was (circle one): Su M T (W) Th F Sat Last night's date: _October 16_

PART I: LAST NIGHT'S SLEEP QUALITY

1. What time did you turn out the light and try to sleep last night?
___10:50___

2. How difficult was it for you to fall asleep? (Circle one.)

        (1)   2   3   4   5
  Not very difficult   Extremely difficult

3. How many times did you awaken during the night? _None_

4. Record how many minutes you were awake for each awakening you listed above in question 3. _____ _____ _____

5. What is the last time you awakened this morning?_____What is the total time you slept last night? _7_ hours, _45_ minutes.

6. How rested do you feel this morning? (Circle one.)

        (1)   2   3   4   5
   Very rested   Poorly rested

7. Rate the overall quality of last night's sleep. (Circle one.)

        1   (2)   3   4   5
   Excellent   Very poor

PART II: BEHAVIOR YESTERDAY AND LAST NIGHT

8. If you napped yesterday: When? _____ For how long? _____

9. For each of the variables you monitered, describe what occurred yesterday.   Low   High

Variable 1 (Variable: _Exercise_) Rating if appropriate: (1) 2 3 4 5
Observation: _None all day_

                         Low   High
Variable 2 (Variable: _Alcohol use_) Rating if appropriate: 1 2 3 4 5
Observation: _One glass of wine with dinner_

                         Low   High
Variable 3 (Variable: _Bedtime snack_) Rating if appropriate: 1 2 3 4 5
Observation: _Popcorn an hour before bed_

                         Low   High
Variable 4 (Variable: _Job stress_) Rating if appropriate: (1) 2 3 4 5
Observation: _A good day. Developed good case strategies with client_

Figure 4-2

Ms. Frazier's Sleep Log on the Best Night (Wednesday)

DAILY SLEEP LOG

Name __Judy Frazier__

Last night was (circle one): Su M T W Th (F) Sat   Last night's date: _October 18_

PART I: LAST NIGHT'S SLEEP QUALITY

1. What time did you turn out the light and try to sleep last night?
   __10:45__

2. How difficult was it for you to fall asleep? (Circle one.)
   (1)   2   3   4   5
   Not very difficult   Extremely difficult

3. How many times did you awaken during the night? __3__

4. Record how many minutes you were awake for each awakening
   you listed above in question 3. __90__   __40__   __15__

5. What is the last time you awakened this morning? _6:30_ What is
   the total time you slept last night? __5__ hours, __20__ minutes.

6. How rested do you feel this morning? (Circle one.)
   1   2   3   (4)   5
   Very rested   Poorly rested

7. Rate the overall quality of last night's sleep. (Circle one.)
   1   2   3   4   (5)
   Excellent   Very poor

PART II: BEHAVIOR YESTERDAY AND LAST NIGHT

8. If you napped yesterday: When? _____ For how long? _____

9. For each of the variables you monitered, describe what occurred
   yesterday.   Low   High

Variable 1 (Variable: _Exercise_) Rating if appropriate: 1 2 3 4 (5)
Observation: _Worked out at the rec center for 25 minutes after work_
                                         Low   High
Variable 2 (Variable: _Alcohol use_) Rating if appropriate: 1 2 3 4 5
Observation: _1 glass of wine with dinner. 1 more at 10:00, to celebrate weekend_
                                         Low   High
Variable 3 (Variable: _Bedtime snack_) Rating if appropriate: 1 2 3 4 5
Observation: _Granola bar and milk just before bed_
                                         Low   High
Variable 4 (Variable: _Job stress_) Rating if appropriate: 1 2 3 4 (5)
Observation: _Judge denied our motion, so brief is due next week_

Figure 4-3

Ms. Frazier's Sleep Log on the Worst Night (Friday)

she thought that her best night of sleep was Wednesday. That was the only night that hadn't been interrupted with nighttime awakenings. The worst nights were Tuesday and Friday, when she had long awakenings.

The next thing Ms. Frazier did was to scrutinize the information she had recorded on her sleep log regarding the four variables predicted to affect sleep. One variable at a time, she examined what had been going on with each of the four variables during the days and evenings preceding the one good and two bad sleep nights.

She found that the first variable — daytime or evening exercise — did not seem to correlate with the quality of sleep on those nights. As you see on the sleep logs, she exercised on Friday afternoon, the day before a bad night's sleep, and she didn't exercise on Wednesday, the day before the best night's sleep. Based on these observations, she concluded that daytime exercise did not significantly affect the quality of her nighttime sleep. She decided that there was no further need to monitor this variable after the first week.

Ms. Frazier then went to the second variable: alcohol use. She'd had a drink with dinner four evenings during the week, and sleep hadn't always suffered those nights. But she had had a glass of wine *within two hours of bedtime* on both Tuesday and Friday — the two worst nights of sleep. Although she had fallen asleep very quickly on those nights, she was bothered both nights by nighttime awakenings and difficulty returning to sleep.

She recognized a phenomenon that we will explore in Chapter 8: Alcohol often makes it easy to fall asleep, but the sleeper tends to awaken and to stay awake for long periods during the night. She continued monitoring alcohol use for a second week. Based on what Ms. Frazier learned from the sleep log, she decided to limit her alcohol intake to one drink with dinner. (Afterward she found that making this simple change improved her sleep considerably.)

She looked next at the third variable: having a bedtime snack. Here she saw no clear correlation between late-night food and the quality of sleep. For example, you can see that she had a granola bar and milk at bedtime on Friday, her worst sleep night. She stopped monitoring this variable after the first week, because it seemed not to affect the quality of her sleep.

Ms. Frazier then looked at the fourth variable: work-related stress. The information on the sleep log was less clear here. The log showed that the most stressful days at work had been Monday and Friday. Sure enough, she had slept poorly Friday night, but she had already seen that late-night alcohol contributed to awakenings that night. And Monday night's sleep had been just a little worse than her average.

At this point Ms. Frazier wasn't sure if her daytime job stress really did hurt her sleep that night. But she looked again at the sleep logs and saw a possible correlation between the day's job stress and that night's sleeplessness. The correlation wasn't as clear-cut as the one between late-night alcohol and sleeplessness. But there was a general tendency: She seemed to sleep better when job stress had been low that day, and she slept poorly when the job had been especially stressful that day.

Not only that, but she realized that the late-night drink on Tuesday had been *in response to the day's stress.* In other words, job stress had led to the nightcap, which led in turn to nighttime awakenings and the inability to return to sleep. Remember, she had had a nightcap on Friday night, too. The late-evening drink that night had been in part to celebrate the end of the workweek and in part because it had been a rough day. So job stress seemed to cause a sleep problem *indirectly* on each of those nights, by leading to a late-night glass of wine.

Ms. Frazier concluded that job stress *did* appear to contribute to insomnia. She continued for one more week to monitor job stress and nighttime sleep, correlating the two.

After two weeks of self-monitoring, she was certain that daytime job stress contributed to her nighttime sleep problems.

For these reasons, Ms. Frazier decided to investigate techniques for managing daytime and evening stress. She learned stress-reduction exercises, which she did for twenty minutes each day at her lunch hour or after work. She also used relaxation exercises at bedtime on those nights when she felt particularly tense.

With the two steps Ms. Frazier took — cutting out alcohol after dinner and learning stress-management techniques during the daytime — it didn't take her long to begin sleeping more soundly through the night.

YOU ARE YOUR OWN BEST DIAGNOSTICIAN

Many insomnia sufferers who come to sleep disorders centers expect that a sleep therapist will be the person to identify the source of the problem. However, the person with the sleep problem is the one who can best know what sleep-related behaviors to monitor. And that person is the one who can best monitor his or her own behavior.

It's up to you. Nobody knows you as well as you do. You are the one responsible for identifying the variables to monitor in your sleep log. You are the one responsible for monitoring and recording your daytime behavior and nighttime sleep. If you make the effort, you can become your own personal sleep therapist. This will be an important step in overcoming your insomnia and learning to sleep better.

Part III
Solutions for the Eight Major Causes of Insomnia

CHAPTER 2 PRESENTED AN OVERVIEW OF THE DIFFERENT types of sleep disorders, including a brief survey of eight major causes of insomnia. The eight chapters in Part III examine in detail each of those causes:

- *Sleep changes with aging*
- *Medical conditions and medication effects*
- *Sleeping pills*
- *Alcohol, tobacco, and caffeine*
- *Depression*
- *Stress and anxiety*
- *Disordered sleep-wake rhythms*
- *Sleeplessness associated with the bed and bedroom*

You probably don't need to read all these chapters carefully. Focus especially on the chapter or chapters that cover the particular cause or causes of your insomnia that you discovered through your diagnostic work in Chapters 3 and 4.

Be sure to read Chapter 12. It tells what to do about a type of insomnia that can develop as a later consequence of a sleeping problem due to any cause.

5

Sleep Changes with Aging

THIS CHAPTER EXAMINES THE NATURAL CHANGES IN SLEEP that accompany the aging process. It surveys sleep problems common among older adults and reviews recommendations for improving sleep as we grow older. It also discusses ways to keep a good attitude toward the changes in sleep we experience with age.

It is important to know how sleep changes naturally as we grow older. This knowledge can help you determine whether the sleep changes you experience are the normal accompaniments of increasing age, or whether you have a sleep problem that needs intervention.

HOW OUR SLEEP CHANGES AS WE GROW OLDER

There are wide individual differences in how aging affects our sleep, just as in many other aspects of sleep. Some older adults experience changes in sleep at a later age and to a smaller degree than others. However, a few generalizations can be made.

CHANGES IN SLEEP LENGTH

Average daily length of sleep, including naps, declines from seven and a half hours in early adulthood to seven hours by age sixty. By the seventies, it drops to six hours. By age ninety, it drops to five and three quarter hours.

However, this decline in average sleep length does not predict the sleep changes any one person will experience because of individual differences among people. Most adults sleep less as they grow older. But some experience no changes in sleep length with age. And some sleep more than they used to. For example, only 1 percent of thirty-year-olds sleep ten hours or more, but fully 6 percent of seventy-year-olds sleep this long.

CHANGES IN SLEEP QUALITY

If you have reached middle age, you probably have found that you don't sleep as well as you used to. Between age thirty and sixty, most of us notice that we sleep less soundly than before.

Figure 5–1 shows the changes in sleep stages with increasing age. As you can see, time awake in bed and light sleep grow slowly during adulthood, then show a marked increase around age sixty. Conversely, deep sleep declines slowly during adulthood until around the same age, then shows a marked reduction. Remember that the sleep in stages 3 and 4 revitalizes us. Because deep sleep decreases with age, our sleep can feel less refreshing as we grow older.

Let's review what is known about the development of sleep across the human life span.

Figure 5–1
Representation of Changes in Sleep Stages and Sleep Patterns with Increasing Age

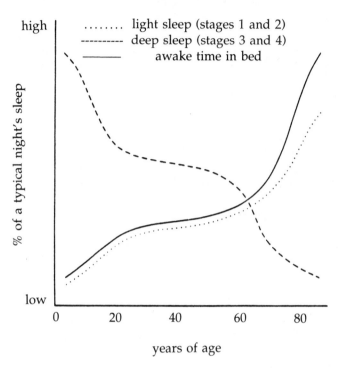

high

.... light sleep (stages 1 and 2)
---------- deep sleep (stages 3 and 4)
———— awake time in bed

% of a typical night's sleep

low

0   20   40   60   80

years of age

From "Insomnia," by Kenneth Lichstein and Suzanne Fischer, in *Handbook of Clinical Behavior Therapy with Adults*, edited by Michael Hersen and Alan Bellack. Copyright © 1985. Reprinted by permission of Plenum Press.

Childhood and Adolescence

During infancy, the wide range of individual differences in sleep behavior first emerges. Although newborn infants average sixteen hours of sleep a day, some may sleep as little as twelve hours and others as much as twenty. We saw in Chapter 1 that genetic factors determine whether a person is a short sleeper or a long sleeper (and Chapter 11 discusses whether someone is a morning person or a night person). We also saw that our genetic endowment predisposes each of us to be a good sleeper or a poor sleeper. Genetically determined individual differences continue to affect sleep during childhood, adolescence, and adulthood.

Early Adulthood (Age Eighteen to Thirty)

Complaints of insomnia are less frequent among young adults than older people. However, significant changes occur in sleep even in early adulthood. During our twenties, the level of deep stage 4 sleep is reduced by half. And by the end of our twenties, we awaken twice as often during the night as we did ten years earlier. Early adulthood is the time in life when some of us first find our sleep disrupted by a snoring bed partner.

Middle Age (Thirty to Sixty)

During middle age, most people notice changes in the quality of their sleep. It may become more difficult to fall asleep. A more common experience is that sleep becomes shallower in depth. Our deepest sleep, stage 4, disappears by age forty. As we age, we also have less of the next-deepest level, stage 3.

We saw in Chapter 2 that a few people appreciate the effects of shallower sleep. Those who experience sleep disorders that occur in deep sleep — sleepwalking and night terrors — find that these problems go away with the loss of deep sleep.

Most people, though, find the developmental sleep changes during middle age to be annoying or distressing. Because our sleep is shallower, we cannot stay asleep as well as we used to. Nighttime awakenings occur three times more often at age sixty than at age twenty. These awakenings are not only more frequent but longer-lasting as well. A period of wakefulness after about three hours of sleep is particularly common.

During middle age, many people become more sedentary. This is important because, as noted in Chapter 14, a lack of exercise can make sleep shallower. Physiological effects of weight gain, another development for some people in middle age, can also disrupt sleep. Chapter 6 explores this problem.

Old Age (Sixty and Older)

The age-related changes in sleep that begin in middle age accelerate toward the end of our life span. The body's most restorative sleep — the deep delta sleep of stages 3 and 4 — declines from 20 or 25 percent of the night's sleep in childhood, to 10 or 15 percent in adulthood, to 5 percent or less in old age. In some older adults, delta sleep is entirely absent.

Because their sleep is shallow, older adults are roused from sleep more easily than younger adults. Older sleepers are more likely to be awakened by external stimuli, such as noises, and by internal arousal signals, such as a full bladder. Frequent awakenings contribute to many older people's observations that their sleep is "lighter" than when they were younger.

Older adults are the most frequent users of sleeping pills. Approximately half of American women and one-fourth of men over age sixty-five occasionally use medications to help them sleep. This is in contrast to about 7 percent of sleeping-pill users in the general adult population.

In old age, some of us become distressed with the developmental changes that make sleep shallower. Dr. J. Allan Hobson, the eminent Harvard University sleep researcher, writes in his thoughtful book *Sleep* (New York: Scientific American Library, 1989) of the difficulty getting deep sleep in old age, suggesting that "at the end we wakefully contemplate the sleep of death with a strange mixture of anxiety, fear, and relief."

However, we need not look negatively on the natural evolution in sleep that accompanies the aging process. Many older adults adapt well to age-related sleep changes. There are several steps you can take to maintain good sleep habits as you grow older, as you will see later in this chapter.

SLEEP PROBLEMS COMMON AMONG OLDER ADULTS

Different surveys show that approximately half of all people over age sixty-five experience insomnia. Sleep-related complaints are the second most frequent reason for older people's visits to physicians. (The most frequent reason involves symptoms of upper respiratory infections.)

All the sleep-disrupting factors discussed in the next seven chapters can operate for adults at any age.

Because older people can have insomnia from any combination of causes, it is important not to attribute your sleep problem automatically to the aging process. Regardless of your age, the most effective way to overcome insomnia is to examine all the behaviors that may affect the quality of your sleep. This is the process of diagnosing your insomnia introduced in Part II. For older adults, just as for younger people, insomnia problems with different causes require different solutions.

In particular, many physiological factors that disrupt sleep are more likely to operate in older adults. As we age, we become more susceptible to the sleep-disrupting effects of caffeine. Diseases that interfere with sleep — such as arthritis, bladder problems, sleep apnea, and restless legs syndrome — affect a greater number of older people than younger ones. With increasing age, medications are metabolized more slowly. For example, a sleeping pill that formerly was metabolized adequately overnight may now remain in the system much longer, causing daytime sedation. Because of these kinds of problems, you may want to read Chapter 6 carefully.

About one-third of adults over sixty-five tend to fall asleep too early in the evening and consequently awaken long before dawn. Another sleep problem found among older adults is that day and night tend to blend together, with increased drowsiness during the day and increased wakefulness during the night. Chapter 11 discusses how to cope with these sleep problems.

RECOMMENDATIONS TO IMPROVE SLEEP FOR OLDER ADULTS

When you try to improve the quality of your sleep, keep two facts in mind. First, you may need to modify your expectations about how well you sleep at night. There are many things that older people cannot do as well as they did when they were younger. Just as it is normal for a sixty-year-old to run less fast and far than a twenty-year-old, it is natural for an older adult to sleep less deeply and soundly than a younger one.

The second fact to remember is that older people are not exempt from any of the factors that cause insomnia in younger adults. It is important for all people with sleep problems, regardless of their ages, to examine their behavior during the day and evening for factors that may interfere with nighttime sleep.

There are several steps that older adults can take that will improve the quality of their sleep in nearly all instances:

1. Because there may not be any pressing reason to get out of bed, it can be tempting to stay in bed late on a morning after you haven't slept well. However, to keep your sleep-wake rhythm regular and encourage sleep the next night, it is important to get out of bed at the same time each day. Don't linger in bed in the morning.

2. Some people experience nighttime sleep problems in old age because they don't keep busy during the day. Become as involved as you can in some kind of regular avocation. Investigate community activities. Ask senior citizens' organizations in your area about social events or groups you can join. Perhaps you can volunteer to help each morning at a local school or day-care center. Cultivate a hobby. Use your imagination to figure out how you can fill up your days with activities you will look forward to.

3. For most people, avoiding naps during the day is the best way to induce sound sleep at night. However, some older adults adapt well to a regular daytime nap. Experiment with naps to see if they are right for you.

    If you nap during the day, it is best to nap before 3:00 P.M. and for no longer than an hour. You should anticipate that your nighttime sleep will be reduced by about the amount of time you nap, so don't expect to nap during the day and then get a full night's sleep.

4. We have seen that nighttime awakening is frequently a problem after middle age. When you awaken during the night, don't *try* to fall back to sleep. Instead just lie in bed for a while to see if sleep returns. Don't watch the clock or think about how long you've been awake. If it seems clear that you won't return to sleep soon — after fifteen or twenty minutes — then do something else. Switch on the light and read, or get up and go to another room. Watch TV, write a letter, do a chore such as cleaning out a drawer, or engage in a quiet hobby until you become drowsy. Then return to bed. If you can't fall asleep, get up and start your day.

    The recommendation to leave the bedroom when you can't sleep is particularly important if you have learned to associate your bed and bedroom with sleeplessness rather than sleep. We will examine this phenomenon in Chapter 12.

5. For those nights when you awaken and can't get back to sleep, develop a menu of activities from which to choose. Consider VCR tapes, projects, and books. Many older adults always have a novel, biography, or some other nonfiction that they look forward to reading when they wake up at night.

   Others have signed up with SeniorNet, a national computer network for people fifty-five and over. When they awaken between midnight and dawn — or at any time of the day — they log onto the network and join lively discussions with other seniors. Topics range from gardening to grandparenting, from health problems to hiking. The network can be accessed any time. There are "cocktail parties" each evening with group chatter and jokes. For many people, this computer network fills a social need and helps them stay active and informed.

   Don't buy the myth about older people being technology-phobic. As this book goes to press, more than fifteen thousand older adults have joined SeniorNet. Others use computers to write regular newsletters for relatives, including such subjects as book reviews and installments of their autobiographies. Go ahead and give it a try; you're only old once.

6. See Chapter 11 for more about how the body's sleep-wake rhythm changes during old age and how to cope with these changes.

   Stay awake until at least 10:00 or 11:00 P.M. to avoid awakening in the hours before dawn. If you get drowsy earlier, take a brisk walk or do some indoor exercise. Try to schedule social contact during the evenings. If you live alone and can't easily socialize with others, you can use radio talk shows or TV programs as a kind of surrogate social group.

7. Don't take sleeping pills on a regular basis, because regular use will probably worsen your sleep problem. If you take sleep medication occasionally or regularly, read Chapter 7 for guidelines concerning when and how to use it.

8. As we grow older, we all must learn to cope with our own aging, chronic illness, the deaths of friends, and the prospect of death for ourselves. If you are preoccupied with any of these issues — or any distressing emotional problem — examine Chapters 9 and 10, which include self-help techniques for troubling emotions, as well as guidelines for when and how to seek professional help.

9. Use the techniques in Part IV that have helped people of all ages improve the quality of their sleep.

KEEP A GOOD ATTITUDE TOWARD SLEEP

As you age, you may experience more difficulty falling asleep than when you were younger. Probably you will awaken more often during the night and sleep less deeply. It is important to know the facts about sleep and aging, so that you realize the age-related changes in your sleep are normal.

Distress over insomnia is not a necessary part of human development. Accept the fact that it is natural to sleep less well in old age than when you were younger. Abolish habits that keep you from getting the soundest sleep of which you are capable. Take actions to improve the quality of your sleep, and you will feel the quality of your life improve.

Make the effort to learn positive attitudes and habits toward sleep, and you will look forward to bedtime rather than dread it.

6

Medical Conditions and Medication Effects

AS NOTED IN CHAPTER 2, INSOMNIA OFTEN IS A BEHAVIORAL disorder that is caused and maintained by a set of maladaptive habits. But it can also be a symptom of many different medical conditions. To complicate the picture further, insomnia is a side effect of many medications.

In this chapter you will learn how medical problems and medications can affect sleep. If you suspect one of these factors may be influencing your sleep, you should discuss it with your doctor.

MEDICAL CONDITIONS THAT AFFECT SLEEP

Disorders of every organ system in the body can lead to insomnia. Many illnesses have symptoms — such as pain, itch, or shortness of breath — that may be hardly noticeable during the day but interfere with sleep at night. Let's look at some physical conditions that disrupt sleep.

CARDIOVASCULAR DISORDERS

Angina is a condition in which the heart muscle receives insufficient oxygen. The angina sufferer awakens with choking pain during an attack. Nighttime angina attacks are particularly apt to occur during REM sleep. Some sleep experts speculate that angina attacks may be a response to the emotional content of dreams in the REM phase.

Coronary artery disease and *hypertension,* or high blood pressure, can also produce insomnia. Diuretics prescribed for hypertension can cause frequent arousals at night to urinate.

RESPIRATORY DISORDERS

Such conditions as *asthma, bronchitis,* and *emphysema* can interfere with breathing at night, causing the sleeper to awaken. Allergies can trigger breathing and congestion symptoms that interfere with sleep. In addition, the medications used to treat these conditions are very likely to cause insomnia, as you will see later in this chapter.

Sleep apnea is a sleep-induced respiratory impairment in which breathing is interrupted for ten seconds or longer. An episode ends when reflexes lighten sleep enough to wake the person, who gasps for air and falls asleep again. Apnea episodes can happen as often as several hundred times a night.

The disorder is particularly apt to affect men, and it occurs more often with increasing age. In addition, obesity contributes to sleep apnea. The use of tranquilizers, sleeping pills, and alcohol can worsen the disorder.

Sleep apnea is more common than previously thought. A University of Wisconsin research study published in 1993 in the *New England Journal of Medicine* examined sleep apnea and other respiratory problems among 602 people thirty to sixty years old. It was found that 2 percent of women and 4 percent of men suffer from sleep apnea that causes excessive sleepiness during the day. In addition, 9 percent of women and 24 percent of men in the middle-aged population experience disrupted breathing during sleep that does not cause daytime sleepiness.

There are two types of sleep apnea. In *obstructive apnea*, the upper airway closes because of anatomical problems. In the less common *central apnea*, the brainstem's respiratory center fails to signal the breathing muscles to keep moving.

People with sleep apnea typically are not aware of their nighttime breathing problems, because they don't fully awaken during most episodes. But their sleep is disrupted, and consequently the chief complaint is daytime sleepiness. In some cases apnea sufferers complain about insomnia, because they awaken repeatedly but don't know why.

Most people with sleep apnea have not been diagnosed as having this disorder. A person's bed partner can often detect the condition, by hearing episodes of loud snoring, interrupted by silence for ten seconds or longer, followed by gasps for breath. People who sleep alone can run a tape recorder while they sleep, so they can later listen for signs of disturbed breathing.

If you may have sleep apnea, you need to be evaluated at a sleep disorders center. See Appendix 6, and discuss the problem with your doctor.

A person diagnosed with sleep apnea has two major treatment options: corrective surgery, which can be done if there are certain structural abnormalities in the upper airway, and the procedure called *continuous positive airway pressure* (CPAP). In this more common treatment, the apnea sufferer wears a nasal mask attached to a machine that pumps air at slightly above room pressure.

DIGESTIVE DISORDERS

Acid reflux, or *heartburn*, is an inflammation of the esophagus — the food tube from the mouth to the stomach. The esophageal sphincter normally separates the esophagus and the stomach. Heartburn occurs when this sphincter malfunctions and stomach acids back up into the esophagus. Heartburn interferes with sleep because the condition worsens when the person lies down, and in that position stomach acid is more likely to seep into the esophagus, where it triggers a reflex that awakens the sleeper.

If you are susceptible to heartburn, there are several steps you can take to alleviate the problem. Try raising the upper part of your body: Place six-inch blocks beneath the head of the bed, or arrange pillows beneath yourself from your waist to your head. Eat dinner early in the evening, to allow food to be digested before bedtime. Avoid coffee, alcohol, chocolate, and fats, because these substances stimulate acid secretion. Stop smoking, because tobacco smoke weakens the esophageal sphincter that malfunctions in heartburn. Over-the-counter antacids can provide some relief.

An *ulcer* is a lesion that appears in the esophagus, stomach, or intestine. One out of seven people suffers from ulcers. Ulcer patients often experience insomnia caused by the effects of stomach acids that are secreted during sleep. While the stomachs of most people secrete less acid during sleep than during the day, the stomachs of ulcer patients secrete much more acid during asleep.

BLADDER PROBLEMS

Some people, particularly in old age, suffer disrupted sleep because of the frequent need to urinate at night. Their bladder problems cause them to awaken, and then they have a hard time falling back asleep.

Frequent urination during the day or night is often caused by excessive caffeine use (see Chapter 8). If you use caffeine, try doing without it for a few days to see if the condition improves. If avoiding caffeine doesn't help, or if you don't use caffeine, see your physician. He or she may recommend that you retrain your urinary reflexes.

You can retrain your reflexes by progressively delaying

urination each time you feel the urge during the day and evening. During the first week, whenever you feel the need to urinate, try to delay using the bathroom for fifteen minutes. In the second week, increase the interval between urge and urination to thirty minutes. Try to add fifteen minutes to the interval each week, until you have increased it to ninety minutes by the sixth week.

After you are able to delay urination for ninety minutes, the next step is to increase the amount of water you drink, to strengthen your urinary reflex further. Drink an extra glass of water each morning for a week, and add another glass each week, until after a month you are drinking four glasses — or about a quart — each morning.

You may want to restrict fluids in the evenings. If you do, be careful to avoid dehydration.

Retraining the urinary reflex solves the problem of frequent nighttime urination for most people. However, women who tend to develop yeast infections and men with prostate problems may not be good candidates for this method. They should discuss alternate treatment approaches with their physicians.

MUSCULOSKELETAL DISORDERS

Pain and stiffness of *arthritis* and *other rheumatic disorders* can keep people awake at night. Sleep may be disrupted when a person with arthritis rolls over and upsets an inflamed joint.

Some people seem to sleep well at night but awaken in the morning feeling tired. Their sleep seems not to refresh them. They experience general malaise, with no particular area of pain. A person who experiences localized tenderness and widespread musculoskeletal stiffness — similar to what arthritis sufferers feel — may be suffering from *fibrositis*. This disease produces subtle symptoms similar to arthritis, along with fatigue, mood disturbance, and sleep that is restless and nonrestorative. Sometimes medication helps reduce the severity of this problem.

MOVEMENT DISORDERS

As many as 5 to 10 percent of adults experience involuntary body movements at night. Either or both of two major disorders can occur.

The term "periodic limb movements" describes a condition in which the person's legs — or, less often, the arms — twitch uncontrollably for a few seconds. These twitches tend to occur periodically every twenty to thirty seconds. An episode may last from a few minutes to a few hours or even longer. If it awakens a sleeper, that person, not knowing the cause of the awakening, will likely complain of insomnia. If the disorder disturbs sleep without full awakening, the person will likely complain of excessive daytime sleepiness.

Periodic limb movements become more common with age. The condition sometimes is treated with muscle-relaxing drugs, such as Valium. However, it is easy to become addicted to these kinds of medications. Other types of medications can help reduce periodic limb movements in some instances. In cases where poor peripheral blood circulation is involved, vitamin E supplements or a warm bath before bedtime may reduce the symptoms.

Restless legs syndrome is a phenomenon in which the person experiences unpleasant sensations in the legs while lying down. These sensations have been compared to crawling flesh or to feeling ants walking around inside the legs. The sensations occur mainly in the calves, but they may also affect the thighs and feet. They cause strong urges to move the legs by shaking them, massaging them, or getting up and walking around.

The sensations most often occur while the person is falling asleep, causing sleep-onset insomnia. In some instances, though, sensations appear during the night, awakening the person. Symptoms disappear when the person gets out of bed but recur when he or she lies down again.

Research suggests that people with restless legs syndrome have a genetic predisposition to the disorder. Various kinds of medication therapies — Clonopin, Restoril, Tegretol, B vitamins — can decrease the severity of the condition.

Periodic limb movements and restless legs syndrome should not be confused with nocturnal leg cramps. Although leg cramps can be quite painful, they rarely indicate a serious medical problem. They usually are a delayed reaction to strenuous daytime activity, but they can also be caused by inactivity. If you experience nighttime leg cramps, try adjusting your daytime activity level one way or the other. Daily calf-stretching exercises just before bedtime can help prevent leg cramps. If you experience a cramp, try to interrupt it immediately by stretching your leg out straight and bending your toes back toward your head.

Periodic limb movements and restless legs syndrome are also different from sudden jerks of the whole body that occur sometimes at sleep onset. These body jerks sometimes are accompanied by a mental image such as missing a step. They are normal responses unrelated to movement disorders.

EPILEPSY

People with epileptic conditions experience a rate of insomnia twice that of the general population. Some epileptics are particularly subject to sleepwalking and night terrors.

PREGNANCY

Women usually experience daytime sleepiness during pregnancy, especially during the first few months. This sleepiness may be due to an increase in the hormone progesterone, which has a sedating effect.

In the second trimester of pregnancy, daytime sleepiness

diminishes or disappears. But in the last trimester, a pregnant woman often has difficulty falling asleep and staying asleep. She doesn't sleep well because of body discomfort related to the position or movements of the fetus.

Sleep medications can harm the fetus of a pregnant woman. A safe alternative is to follow the sleep-inducing procedures in Chapters 14 and 15.

MENOPAUSE

Many women experience increased difficulty with sleep when they reach menopause. Restless sleeping and early-morning awakenings are particularly common.

Estrogen replacement can improve the sleep quality of menopausal women. However, there are significant medical risks associated with this treatment. A woman contemplating estrogen replacement needs to discuss with her gynecologist the potential risks and benefits.

OTHER MEDICAL CONDITIONS

It is obvious how any of the above disorders can lead directly to insomnia. However, some other kinds of medical problems can interfere with sleep in more subtle ways. These include the *Epstein-Barr virus, hyperthyroidism,* kidney disorders such as *uremia,* and endocrine disorders such as *diabetes.* A thorough discussion with your doctor is in order if you suspect one of these disorders may be interfering with your sleep.

EFFECTS OF DRUGS ON SLEEP

PRESCRIPTION AND OVER-THE-COUNTER MEDICATIONS

Many different classes of prescription and nonprescription medication may cause poor sleep. If you need to take a certain type of medication, you may have little choice. In most instances, though, you can arrange a modified treatment with your doctor. You may be able to alter the dosage strength or the time you take the medication. Your physician also may consider switching to a related drug, so that your medical condition can be treated without causing insomnia as a side effect. For example, the antidepressant Vivactil can interfere with sleep, in contrast with the antidepressant Elavil, which is more likely to cause drowsiness at bedtime.

If you are uncertain whether any medication contains sleep-disrupting ingredients, such as caffeine or amphetamine, read the required label on over-the-counter medications or the package insert with prescription drugs. Or ask your pharmacist or doctor.

Listed below are common types of drugs and drug ingredients that can cause insomnia:

- *Drugs containing caffeine, such as Excedrin, Anacin, or Triaminicin*

- *Drugs containing amphetamine, such as prescription diet pills*

- *Drugs containing adrenocorticotropic hormone (ACTH), such as Acthar*

- *Beta blockers, particularly propranolol (Inderal)*

- *Nasal decongestants*

- *Bronchodilating drugs for asthma*

- *Drugs to control high blood pressure*

- *Drugs to control Parkinsonism*

- *Certain antidepressant drugs*

- *Steroid preparations*

- *Thyroid hormones*

- *Some cancer chemotherapeutic agents*
- *Oral contraceptives*
- *Antimetabolites*
- *Sleeping pills and tranquilizers*

You may be surprised to see sleeping pills and tranquilizers on a list of insomnia-causing drugs. With these kinds of drugs, insomnia can result from withdrawal on nights when you don't use them. We will examine this problem in Chapter 7.

The drugs listed above can cause both major types of insomnia — difficulty falling asleep and difficulty staying asleep.

ASPIRIN

For some people, taking two aspirin (650 mg) at bedtime reduces awakenings during the second half of the night. However, aspirin also reduces the deep sleep of stages 3 and 4 and correspondingly increases shallower stage 2 sleep. Because aspirin reduces nighttime awakenings, it can be helpful in giving relief if you are disturbed by waking during the night. But because aspirin can also make sleep shallower, it may be best not to use it when you need to feel refreshed and restored the next day.

Taking aspirin more than two nights a week diminishes its effect of reducing nighttime awakenings. So if you take aspirin at bedtime to help you sleep through the night, use it no more often than twice a week. Be sure to consult your physician first if you have problems with ulcers or with intestinal or bleeding disorders or — as with any drug — if you are pregnant or nursing a child.

ALCOHOL

Many people use alcohol to induce sleep. In fact, this drug usually does quicken sleep onset initially. However, many people soon develop tolerance to alcohol's sleep-inducing effects, so that before long the drug no longer brings on sleep.

More significantly, alcohol disrupts sleep by causing awakenings during the night. Chapter 8 examines in detail its effects on sleep.

MARIJUANA

Marijuana, or cannabis, is a pharmaceutical enigma. It is neither a stimulant nor a depressant, although it has features of both. Marijuana contains more than sixty chemical compounds that are unique to the plant, including *tetrahydrocannabinol*, or THC, the major psychoactive ingredient. These compounds, known as *cannabinoids*, are present in various combinations among different varieties of marijuana. Some varieties are more likely than others to produce sedating effects.

In addition to differences in stimulation or sedation among varieties of marijuana, effects of the drug vary widely from one to another. Some users find that it stimulates them and keeps them awake. Others believe that it helps them fall asleep. Still others say that it stimulates them at first, leading to compensatory feelings of relaxation and drowsiness a few hours afterward.

Beginning in 1966, researchers have examined the effects of marijuana on human behavior, including sleep. Despite the difficulty of predicting this drug's sleep effects on any given individual, consistent findings have emerged from studying groups of people. These findings have been obtained in two ways: through surveys of marijuana users, and through controlled research in which subjects were given marijuana in the evening and their sleep was subsequently measured.

Marijuana users have responded to surveys about their own observations of the drug's effects on sleep. For example, in 1971 the *Journal of the American Medical Association* reported the results of structured interviews by psychiatrists of one hundred adult regular marijuana users. Respondents had each used the drug on at least fifty occasions over at least a six-month interval. They were questioned about 105 possible marijuana effects. The authors concluded: "No unpleasant effects were noted as usual occurrences by a majority of subjects. A clear mind, more restful sleep, and a calm feeling after intoxication effects had worn off were reported as usual by a majority."

In addition to subjective surveys, scientific experiments have investigated the effects of marijuana on sleep. In the 1980 *Annual Review of Pharmacology and Toxicology*, a major research article examined medically therapeutic actions of marijuana. This review was written by Louis Lemberger, Ph.D., M.D., professor of pharmacology, medicine, and psychiatry at the University of Indiana and director of clinical pharmacology for Eli Lilly Research Laboratories. Dr. Lemberger stated: "When clinical studies were conducted with marijuana and Δ^9-THC, it was apparent to trained observers that these drugs did produce some degree of relaxation and had sedative-hypnotic [calming and sleep-inducing] activity in healthy volunteers."

Two major effects of marijuana on sleep have been documented. First, it diminishes the amount of time subjects spend in REM sleep. Because REM sleep appears to play a role in consolidating learning and memory, reduced REM may interfere with these processes.

The second major effect of marijuana use is to increase the amount of time subjects spend in deep stage 4 sleep. Two experiments have found this effect to persist as long as subjects were studied, up to twenty nights. However, one study found that deep sleep increased initially, but after four consecutive nights of marijuana use, it began decreasing, until by the eighth night it was below the original baseline level. Because of contradictory evidence, no clear conclusions can be drawn at this time regarding marijuana's long-term effects on deep sleep.

When subjects stop taking marijuana after a long period of regular use, they often report sleep problems for up to a few nights. They take longer to fall asleep, and they get less deep stage 4 sleep. In addition, they often experience the strange and vivid dreams of REM rebound. As Chapter 2 notes, after people have discontinued long-term use of REM-suppressing drugs, they temporarily tend to have dreams that are bizarre and sometimes nightmarish. REM-suppressing drugs include not only marijuana, but also some antidepressant medications.

Like marijuana, tranquilizers and sleeping pills can suppress REM. However, their more significant side effect is to suppress deep sleep. With these drugs, the major withdrawal symptom is not REM rebound but rather rebound insomnia, as you will see in the next chapter.

7
Sleeping Pills

SURPRISINGLY, SLEEP MEDICATIONS CAN MAKE AN INSOMNIA problem worse. The short-term cure sometimes turns into long-term dependence. This chapter reviews four aspects of sleeping pills:

- *Different types of sleeping pills*
- *Problems with using sleep medications*
- *Breaking the sleeping-pill habit*
- *Recommendations for using sleep medication wisely*

Prescription sleeping pills are used by about 4 percent of American adults. Another 3 percent use over-the-counter sleeping pills.

Sleep medications are also known as *hypnotics,* from the Greek god of sleep, Hypnos. Interestingly, this god was depicted pouring slumber from a cornucopia and holding a poppy stalk, the source of the slumber potion. This shows the long human interest in controlling sleep by ingesting substances.

People often refer to hypnotics as sedatives, but there is a difference: Sedation is not sleep. A physician may prescribe a sedative to calm an overwrought person without making him or her sleepy. A sedative given at a higher dose tends to put a person to sleep. Some drugs can be a sedative at a low dose, a hypnotic at a high dose, and an anesthetic at an even higher dose.

DIFFERENT TYPES OF SLEEP MEDICATIONS

An important way that sleep medications differ is by their duration of action. This is measured by *elimination half-life*, which refers to the time it takes for the body to eliminate half of the drug. For example, if a drug has a half-life of six hours, half would be gone in six hours; half of the *remainder* in the body would be gone in another six hours, so that after twelve hours, three-fourths of the drug would be eliminated, and so on.

Older adults require more time than younger adults to eliminate drugs from the body. For this reason, older adults need to use special caution when taking a sleep medication with a relatively long elimination half-life.

BENZODIAZEPINES

For the past twenty years, the benzodiazepines (BZDs) have been physicians' treatment of choice when prescribing sleep medication. This class of fifteen drugs includes the common sedatives Valium and Xanax. These and other BZDs are sometimes prescribed as sleep aids. However, only the five BZDs described below are currently approved by the Food and Drug Administration (FDA) for treating insomnia.

The BZDs are listed in order of their duration of action, from relatively short-acting drugs to longer-lasting ones.

Halcion

Halcion is the brand name of the drug triazolam. It has a fast elimination rate, with a half-life of about two and a half hours. Because of its short duration of action, this drug sometimes runs its course before the night is over, causing early-morning awakening. It is most useful for insomnia that involves difficulty falling asleep. Its fast elimination rate causes less daytime sedation than other BZDs.

In the early 1990s, controversy appeared concerning possible side effects of Halcion, including suicidal and aggressive behavior. In 1991, approval for use of the drug was revoked in Great Britain. In 1992, an FDA advisory committee decided to keep the drug on the market in the United States, but at a lower dosage than previously recommended.

Restoril

This is the brand name of the drug temazepam. It has an average elimination half-life of ten hours. Because of its longer duration of action, it can remain effective throughout the night, and it is often prescribed for people who experience difficulty staying asleep.

ProSom

This drug has an elimination half-life that ranges from ten to twenty-four hours. It is usually prescribed for people who experience nighttime awakening. Because of its long duration of action, ProSom, or estazolam, may cause sedation on the day after taking it.

Doral

Doral, or quazepam, is used most often for insomnia that involves difficulty staying asleep. It has a long elimination half-life, averaging thirty-nine hours. Consequently, its sedating effects are felt well into the following day. Doral is particularly helpful when daytime sedation is desired for people who experience daytime anxiety as well as nighttime insomnia.

Dalmane

This is the brand name of the drug flurazepam. It is most helpful for preventing nighttime awakening. Its elimination half-life ranges from forty to one hundred hours or longer, so its effects are felt strongly during the next day. Dalmane is prescribed to induce daytime sedation as well as for its hypnotic properties.

A NEW SLEEPING PILL

Just before this book went to press, the FDA approved a new type of sleep medication. The drug, zolpidem tartrate, will be sold under the brand name Ambien. It is unrelated to the BZDs and to other sleep medications.

Ambien is eliminated rapidly from the body, with an average half-life of about two and a half hours. Because of its fast elimination rate, it appears to be more suitable for insomnia that involves difficulty with falling asleep than for problems with staying asleep.

Preliminary studies suggest that unlike the BZDs, Ambien does not decrease deep sleep. According to the drug's manufacturer, it is less likely to cause tolerance than are the BZDs.

OLDER TYPES OF PRESCRIPTION SLEEPING PILLS

Barbiturates

Barbiturates were often used in the past to treat insomnia. This class of drugs includes Nembutal, Seconal, and phenobarbital. Barbiturates are viewed now as less desirable for a number of reasons. These powerful drugs have a small margin of safety between the usual dose and a dangerous one; Marilyn Monroe and Jimi Hendrix died of barbiturate overdoses. Barbiturates more often produce side effects, and tolerance to them develops quickly.

A few physicians reportedly continue by habit to prescribe the barbiturates for sleep problems, because they were the drug treatment of choice for insomnia until the BZDs were introduced in 1970. However, they are rarely, if ever, appropriate for treating insomnia.

Placidyl

This drug is unrelated to other sleep medications. Usually it is effective for only a few days at a time.

Chloral Hydrate

This drug is particularly apt to cause serious side effects. It is prescribed for people unable to take other kinds of sleep medications. Chloral hydrate mixed with alcohol produced the knockout drink known as a Mickey Finn.

ANTIDEPRESSANTS

As the name indicates, antidepressant medications were developed to treat depression. They also are very effective in helping some people to sleep. Antidepressants are more likely to cause problems with overdose or drug interactions than the BZDs are, but they are less likely than BZDs to lead to addiction. Side effects of antidepressants may include increased heart rate, dry mouth, and sedation.

OVER-THE-COUNTER SLEEPING PILLS

Nonprescription sleep medications utilize antihistamines as active ingredients. Ironically, the drowsiness caused by antihistamines is actually a side effect of their intended purpose of counteracting allergic symptoms. Like prescription sleep medications, over-the-counter sleeping pills lose effectiveness if taken regularly for long periods.

PROBLEMS WITH REGULAR LONG-TERM USE

Although there are large differences among sleep medications, they all have potential problems and dangers if they are used too often for too long.

POOR-QUALITY SLEEP

Sleep medication can diminish the deep sleep of stages 3 and 4, and correspondingly increase shallower stage 2 sleep. When a person sleeps less deeply, that night's sleep will be less refreshing than natural sleep without drugs. Shallow sleep caused by sleeping pills also may lead to more periods of wakefulness during the night.

IMPAIRED PERFORMANCE THE NEXT DAY

The sedating effects of sleep medication can persist into the next day. Research that has investigated performance on mental tasks (such as learning and decision making) and on motor tasks (such as driving a car) on days after the use of sleeping pills finds that people usually do worse after taking a pill than they do after a night of insomnia. Insomnia can make you feel lethargic or sleepy the next day, but the hangover effect from a sleeping pill can make you feel even worse.

Sleeping pills impair performance the next day because a portion of the sleep medication remains in the body after the night has passed. As we have seen, some medications are better than others at minimizing impaired performance the next day.

SIDE EFFECTS

Sleeping pills cause you to breathe more slowly and shallowly than usual. In most cases this side effect is not significant, but it may greatly disrupt the night's sleep of a person with sleep apnea or another sleep-related respiratory disorder.

Other side effects of sleeping pills include anxiety, dizziness, restlessness, confusion, amnesia, blurred vision, nausea, digestive upset, and frequent urination.

INTERACTION WITH OTHER DRUGS

Sleeping pills slow the activity of the central nervous system. If someone uses a sleeping pill while taking another nervous-system depressant — such as antihistamines, tranquilizers, and alcohol — the effects of the sleep medication will be compounded. To add to this slowing of the body's basic functions, such as breathing, can be dangerous or even fatal. About one-third of drug-related deaths involve sleeping pills.

DANGERS FOR PREGNANT WOMEN

You probably have heard of the birth defects experienced by children born to women who took thalidomide when pregnant. What you may not know is that this drug was used as a sleeping pill.

Any sedative drug, such as alcohol or sleep medication,

has the potential to harm a fetus. And even after birth, a breast-feeding mother may transfer medications to the baby through her milk. A pregnant or breast-feeding woman should discuss with her physician the possible dangers of any drug she takes.

LOSS OF EFFECTIVENESS OVER TIME

Sleeping pills work for only a relatively short while. The older barbiturate forms of sleep medications typically lose effectiveness after one week of nightly use. Newer forms of sleep medications may remain effective for longer, but regular use for two to six weeks can lead to *tolerance*. Drug tolerance means that continuing the initial dose will produce diminished effects, and progressively larger doses are needed to maintain the original effect.

POTENTIAL FOR DEPENDENCE

The two hallmarks of drug dependence are tolerance, discussed above, and *withdrawal*, which refers to symptoms that appear when a drug is removed and disappear when the drug is reinstated. Because withdrawal symptoms go away when a person begins using the drug again, many people do just that: give up trying to quit and return to using the substance.

When a person regularly uses sleeping pills for a long period of time and then stops suddenly, the withdrawal symptom that appears is called rebound insomnia, as noted earlier. People who stop taking the pills after their bodies have learned to depend on them for sleep find that quitting causes their insomnia to be much worse than it was before they began taking pills.

Even though sleeping pills lose effectiveness when used regularly for about a month, many people continue taking them each night for much longer because they want to avoid rebound insomnia. In other words, they have to continue taking sleep medication or they will experience worse insomnia than they had before they took any pills. It's no wonder they keep taking the pills.

Some people say that sleeping pills are all that stands between them and insomnia. The cause of the insomnia that led to sleeping pills may have disappeared long before, but their insomnia continues, driven by the tolerance and withdrawal effects of their addiction to the pills.

As we will see, there are circumstances in which the use of sleep medication is appropriate. However, beginning to take sleeping pills can be like the proverbial dilemma of "riding the tiger": Getting on may be easy, but getting off is much more difficult. Use extreme caution with sleep medication if you have ever had problems with dependence — on alcohol or on other drugs, including tobacco and caffeine — because a history of dependence on any drug makes it more likely that you will become dependent on sleep medication.

HOW TO BREAK A SLEEPING-PILL HABIT

As already noted, regular use of sleeping pills for longer than a few weeks will likely lead to drug dependence. Remember, one of the two signs of drug dependence is tolerance. Because of tolerance, the pills don't work as well as they used to. In fact, even if you take high doses every night, you may sleep no better than you did before you started taking sleeping pills, and you'll probably be experiencing daytime side effects that you didn't have before you began using drugs to sleep. When you realize that this is a bad bargain, you may want to kick the habit.

If you are dependent on a drug, when you quit you will experience the second sign of dependence: withdrawal symptoms that appear when a drug is discontinued. These symptoms typically manifest themselves in rebound insomnia for a few nights — and possibly for as long as a few weeks. In most cases, this insomnia will be worse than the insomnia that originally led you to take sleeping pills. Rebound insomnia can take the form of difficulty falling asleep, difficulty staying asleep, or both.

You will be tempted to go back on pills again. *Don't do it*. That will just perpetuate the problem and delay your day of reckoning. And the longer you are dependent on sleeping pills, the harder it is to quit.

You may experience withdrawal symptoms other than rebound insomnia when you quit. These can include anxiety, depression, fatigue, cramps, nausea, and headache. It won't be fun. But your freedom from pills will be worth the temporary discomfort.

When you know you are ready to quit taking sleeping pills, follow these guidelines:

1. Ask for advice from the physician who prescribed the medication because he or she knows your medical history and the circumstances surrounding your drug use. If you don't feel confident in your doctor or if you want a second opinion, see another physician.
2. Choose a specific time of at least four weeks to go through the withdrawal symptoms you can expect when you quit. Some people prefer to quit on a vacation or at some other time with reduced demands. Others prefer to go through the stress of withdrawal during a time that is stressful anyway.
3. Emotional support will be helpful during what will likely be a difficult process. Consider meeting regularly with your doctor or a mental-health professional during the withdrawal time. You also can tell someone close to you about your plan to quit using sleeping pills. This will provide you with a source of emotional support and an additional incentive to stick to your intention of quitting.
4. Withdraw gradually rather than cold turkey. During the first week cut your usual dosage by a fourth. Cut

the dosage by another fourth during each of the next two weeks.

If you are taking tablets, cut the pills with a sharp knife. If you are taking capsules, ask your doctor or pharmacist about the advisability of opening the capsule and removing a portion of the contents.

5. Lay in a supply of books, VCR tapes, or hobby materials to keep you busy through the sleepless nights you can expect during the withdrawal period.
6. When you feel anxious about losing sleep without pills, remember what you learned in Chapter 1: Sleeping less at night won't harm your health or your daytime performance.
7. Keep up with exercise, relaxation, and the other sleep aids presented in Chapters 14 and 15.
8. When you finish the withdrawal process, have a celebration, and flush away any pills you have left.

In some instances of extreme addiction, a person must be hospitalized for a week or more to get through the withdrawal process. However, in most cases withdrawal can be undergone safely in a person's home and workplace with the support of a physician or mental-health professional.

RECOMMENDATIONS FOR USING SLEEP MEDICATION WISELY

Sleep medications don't really improve sleep; as we have seen, they make sleep shallower rather than deeper. Their actions *inhibit our ability to stay awake.* If you choose to use sleep medications, remember that they are at best a temporary solution with a potential for significant problems.

Many people have learned to use sleeping pills safely. Most sleeping-pill use is accounted for by people who use sleeping pills fewer than thirty times a year. Three out of four users take sleep medication for two weeks or less at a time. In Gallup polls most people say that sleeping pills relieve their sleeplessness, that they use sleeping pills infrequently, and that they would choose to use them again when insomnia recurs.

William Dement, M.D., Ph.D., director of the Stanford University Sleep Disorders Center and one of the nation's foremost sleep researchers, recently wrote in *The Sleepwatchers* (Stanford Alumni Association, 1992), his book about sleep research: "It is my medical opinion that sleeping pills give excellent relief, are typically needed for only a few nights, and should not be irrationally withheld by the physician."

The situation in which the use of sleeping pills may be most appropriate is a temporary emotional crisis that seriously interferes with sleep. For example, after the death of a spouse many people experience severe insomnia.

Using sleep medication in times of crisis may help you prevent a short-term sleeping problem from turning into a chronic one. As we will see in Chapter 12, conditioned insomnia may arise when you associate your bed and bedroom with frustrated wakefulness rather than with sleep. The short-term use of sleep medications can reduce insomnia during a stressful time, preventing you from developing anxiety and poor sleep-related habits that cause insomnia to persist after the stress goes away.

If you choose to use sleep medication, follow these guidelines:

1. Thoroughly discuss with your doctor the available options. Be sure that he or she knows about any medical condition you have that might complicate the use of sleep medication. Make your physician aware of any other prescription or nonprescription medications you are taking, in order to avoid drug interactions. Finally, ask your doctor about side effects, how long he or she expects you to take the medication, and the danger of dependence on the prescribed drug.

2. Ask your doctor or pharmacist how long before bedtime to take the medication, because sleeping pills differ greatly in how quickly they begin working in the body.

3. Use the lowest dose that works for you. If you take sleeping pills to help you sleep in a short-term crisis, stop using them as soon as the situation improves to decrease the probability that you will become addicted to the medication.

4. Don't take a higher dose than your physician has prescribed. If you find that the old dosage no longer works, you may be experiencing drug tolerance. The best thing to do is to discontinue the medication for a month or longer. (See the section of this chapter that tells how to break a sleeping pill habit.)

5. If pain causes sleeplessness, pain medication is preferable to a sleeping pill. If depression causes insomnia, an antidepressant can reduce symptoms of depression and improve sleep as a medication side effect.

6. Some physicians say that if a patient feels unable to sleep, it is all right to take a pill with a fast elimination rate, such as Halcion, as late as 1:00 A.M. Generally, though, it is best not to take a sleeping pill in the middle of the night. If you have problems with staying asleep through the night or with early-morning awakening, it is best to take a longer-acting medication at bedtime rather than take a pill when you awaken during the night.

   Make sure your physician knows whether your major sleep problem is one of falling asleep or staying asleep. Remember, medications with shorter elimination half-lives are better for falling asleep, while those with longer half-lives are better for staying asleep.

7. Be careful about driving or using dangerous machinery the day after you have taken sleep medication.

8. Never drink alcohol or take a sedative if you are using sleeping pills. This combination can be dangerous — even lethal.

9. If you experience significant side effects during the day, discuss with your physician the options regarding a different dosage or a different medication.

10. Physicians disagree about how often to take sleep medications during a short-term crisis. Some recommend taking medication every night, to establish a strong pattern of consistently good sleep. However, most recommend taking medication on an "as needed" basis, no more than two to four nights a week. One variation on this pattern is to take sleep medication only on the third night after two consecutive nights of poor sleep. Discuss this issue with your doctor.

11. Never give a sleeping pill to a child or adolescent, unless a physician prescribed it for that person. If your child has difficulty sleeping, read Appendix 5. Then ask the pediatrician for advice.

12. Use special caution with sleep medication if you are over sixty. The older you are, the longer a sleeping pill will stay in your body. That is, the drug's half-life will be lengthened. In late adulthood, the liver takes longer to break down a drug, and the kidneys are slower to excrete the drug. For this reason, lower doses of sleep medication often are prescribed for older adults than for younger ones.

13. Remember that in all cases of insomnia it is better to change your habits than to take a pill. Review the strategies throughout this book for improving sleep, and learn how to use them to overcome your insomnia.

8

Alcohol, Tobacco, and Caffeine

THREE SUBSTANCES COMMONLY USED IN OUR SOCIETY CAN severely disrupt sleep. Most of us are aware of caffeine's stimulant effects. However, the actions of alcohol and of the nicotine in tobacco can interfere with sleep even more.

This chapter examines how these three drugs affect sleep and reviews ways to limit the sleep problems they cause. You won't be asked to give up a substance you enjoy — with the exception of tobacco. Instead, you will be shown how to modify your drug-consuming habits to improve the quality of your sleep.

ALCOHOL

Physicians used to prescribe a mixed drink or a glass of wine at bedtime as a remedy for insomnia. Many people still believe that a bedtime nip of alcohol will help them sleep — hence the reference to a "nightcap." But alcohol is not a good sleep aid. In fact, alcohol use is estimated to be the major cause of at least 10 percent of chronic insomnia cases.

As noted earlier, most people who drink alcohol as a bedtime sedative do find that it helps them relax enough to drop off to sleep. Some people, however, have a lot of trouble falling asleep after drinking alcohol. This may be because alcohol use can raise the level of noradrenaline, a chemical in the brain that interferes with sleep.

Regardless of its effect at bedtime, the major problem with alcohol involves not falling asleep but staying asleep. As the body metabolizes alcohol, withdrawal effects occur, causing the person to awaken. Even one drink within two hours of bedtime can cause nighttime awakenings and difficulty falling back asleep. Sleep becomes less deep and less sound. Even if alcohol does help a person fall asleep more quickly, there will be less total sleep over the course of the night.

Sleep that is disrupted and shallow is not the only problem caused by nighttime use of alcohol. For some people, alcohol's sedative effect initiates or worsens episodes of sleep apnea, the respiratory disorder reviewed in Chapter 6. Alcohol aggravates breathing problems during sleep because it relaxes throat muscles and interferes with the involuntary mechanisms that control respiration.

The sleep patterns of chronic alcoholics resemble those of people in old age. They get little or no deep delta sleep. Their shallow sleep is disrupted by many awakenings. Their bodies' basic sleep-wake rhythms become blurred, causing daytime sleepiness and nighttime wakefulness. Fortunately, those alcoholics who quit drinking — except for a relatively small number who have had severe long-term habits — eventually experience improved sleep.

People display a wide range of individual differences in their responses to alcohol, just as with most drugs. If you want to determine alcohol's effect on your sleep, include it as one of the variables in your sleep log (Chapter 4). You can then do a simple experiment: Compare your sleep on those nights when you have a drink near bedtime with your sleep on those nights when you don't. Probably you will find that you sleep worse at night and feel worse in the morning after you have had a nightcap.

Using your sleep log, you also can investigate whether alcohol earlier in the evening disrupts your sleep. Some people find that even one drink with dinner makes them sleep badly, while others have problems only if they drink within about two hours of bedtime.

The more you learn about the effects of alcohol on your sleep, the more you will want to cut back on your night-time use of the drug. If you are accustomed to having one or more drinks during the evening, you may have difficulty stopping all at once. For most people it is best to withdraw gradually. Cut back the amount of your alcohol consumption a little at a time. Some people do well by substituting alcohol-free beer or wine for the real thing. Others enjoy drinking beverages such as fruit juice, rather than switching from alcohol directly to water.

If you try to stop drinking after dinner but find you can't, you may need outside help for an addiction problem. Some people feel that Alcoholics Anonymous is a useful source of support. Others undergo counseling with a behavioral therapist who specializes in substance abuse. Some with severe chronic alcoholism need to be hospitalized to go through withdrawal. If you find you can't stop on your own, talk to your physician to help determine the best way to quit.

If you stop drinking alcohol in the evening, your sleep will improve. In most cases improvement comes within a week or two. If you have been drinking heavily for years, it may take longer. As we have seen, in severe cases sleep never recovers entirely from chronic heavy drinking. But your sleep will become better than it was during times of heavy alcohol use.

It is important to note that in some instances withdrawing from alcohol can initially *worsen* a person's insomnia before it improves. And as we have seen with sleeping pills, withdrawal symptoms typically disappear when you return to using the drug. For this reason, there is a danger that when you quit using evening alcohol, temporary withdrawal symptoms of greater sleeplessness may lead you to resume drinking at night. Be aware of this danger, and mobilize your resolve to stick with your plan of limiting alcohol consumption to dinnertime or earlier.

TOBACCO

The nicotine in tobacco is a drug. More specifically, it is a stimulant that affects the heart, blood vessels, nervous system, and other organs. People who ingest nicotine by smoking or chewing tobacco tend to experience both major types of insomnia problems. First, they have difficulty falling asleep because nicotine speeds up heart rate, raises blood pressure, and stimulates brain wave activity. Second, they have difficulty staying asleep because nicotine withdrawal during the night may make them awaken after several hours craving a smoke. Because their sleep is fragmented, smokers get less restorative sleep.

Millions of people have given up the tobacco habit. Although some find it surprisingly easy to quit, for most people it is a difficult undertaking. After you quit, whether it has been relatively easy or difficult for you to give up smoking, you can look forward to no more morning coughs, throat phlegm, or smoker's breath. Food will taste better, your sense of smell will return, your clothes and hair and home will be cleaner, you will save money that used to go up in smoke — *and you will sleep much better.*

There is a wide range of approaches and programs to help people quit smoking, and no single one works best for all smokers. You may want to contact the Lung Association for information on different programs that can help you quit (1740 Broadway, New York, NY 10019; 212-315-8700). Your physician will have information on such nicotine-replacement methods as skin patches, tablets, or gum. While undergoing withdrawal, some people smoke herbal cigarettes as a replacement for tobacco; these are available from health-food stores. You will have a higher likelihood of success if you use an approach you feel comfortable with.

Some people believe that quitting cold turkey is best, to get the withdrawal symptoms over with all at once. Most people, though, find it useful to cut down before quitting, to minimize the severity of withdrawal symptoms by extending the withdrawal period.

If you choose to cut down before you stop, first set the date for quitting. As the date approaches, gradually decrease the number of cigarettes you smoke each day. You can begin by smoking only one cigarette an hour, or you can decide to smoke only every other hour — for example, only from nine to ten o'clock and from eleven o'clock to noon, and so on. Or you can smoke only half of each cigarette. Or switch to a cigarette with a lower nicotine content as you approach quitting day. Any combination of these strategies decreases the amount of nicotine in your body as you prepare to quit, thereby making withdrawal less severe when you stop smoking entirely.

When the day arrives, tell friends about your big change. Their awareness will give you social support and increased motivation to stay off cigarettes.

After you quit, you almost certainly will experience craving for a smoke at times. Here are some ideas for combating the craving:

- *Drink glasses of water frequently.*

- *Nibble fruit, celery, carrots. Chew gum. Gnaw on toothpicks.*

- *Exercise vigorously. (For this reason, some people quit during an active vacation when they swim, play tennis, or hike.)*

- *Stay away from friends who smoke for a few weeks.*

- *Substitute some other activity for a cigarette in high-risk situations. After coffee and meals, try a mouthwash instead of a cigarette, or take a brisk walk around the block.*

- *Remind yourself often of the major health risks inherent in smoking.*

Prepare for the possibility of weight gain. Your appetite will become fresher and stronger, and you may use food as a substitute for nicotine. Some people pamper themselves with good food while they are withdrawing from cigarettes. Others relish the double challenge of controlling their wish for fattening food while they are controlling their wish for cigarettes. Again, do what works best for you.

Prepare for the possibility of relapse. Don't fall for the "saint-or-sinner" trap of thinking that smoking one cigarette makes you a fallen angel. If you have one cigarette, you don't have to begin smoking regularly again. Don't let perfectionist standards cause you to lose sight of the progress you have made. Keep in mind that giving up cigarettes is a difficult process, and remember all the reasons you have for quitting. One of them is that you will fall asleep more easily and sleep more soundly through the night.

You also have to be aware that your sleep may become worse for a few days after you quit smoking. Just as with sleeping pills and alcohol, you can expect temporary insomnia as a predictable part of the drug-withdrawal process when you give up nicotine. Again, have good books or videos on hand for a few sleepless nights. But if you don't let this minor short-term problem stop you, it won't be long before you are sleeping better — and living better — as a nonsmoker.

CAFFEINE

Many people use caffeine as a pick-me-up, in the form of coffee, tea, soda pop, chocolate, or tablets. This drug increases alertness by stimulating the adrenal glands to produce hormones that rush glucose into the bloodstream. Like other stimulants, caffeine disrupts sleep.

Insomnia sufferers often use caffeine to overcome fatigue caused by the previous night's poor sleep. This caffeine consumption in turn can lead to another night of poor sleep, which then leads to more caffeine. The habit of using this drug to cope with insomnia can result in a continuing cycle of caffeine use and sleeplessness.

In general, consuming more than 250 milligrams of caffeine a day (two to three cups of coffee) will worsen a person's sleep as well as lead to caffeine addiction. However, just as with sleeping pills and alcohol, there is a wide range of individual differences in people's responses to caffeine. Some people can tolerate caffeine relatively well, but others experience sleep problems when they have just one morning cup of coffee or midday glass of cola.

Sensitivity to the effects of caffeine increases with age. Even if you were able to use this drug with little effect on your sleep in the past, it may disrupt your sleep as you grow older.

Excessive caffeine consumption not only leads to insomnia but may also cause nervousness, irritability, shaky hands, heart palpitations, nausea, stomach pain, frequent urination, and diarrhea. If you experience any of these symptoms, you may need to reduce your caffeine intake.

Heavy caffeine users suffer withdrawal effects not just when they give it up entirely. Withdrawal effects occur *every day* for those who are addicted to this drug. Studies show that caffeine users are actually groggier than nonusers when they awaken. Caffeine addicts need a dose of the drug each morning to get themselves going, and they continue to need it through the day as the effects of each dose diminish. Because "what goes up must come down," caffeine users find that when the effects of a dose dissipate, they feel less alert than someone who never uses the drug. This occurs first thing in the morning and throughout the

Item	Average Milligrams of Caffeine
Coffee (5-ounce cup)	
Brewed by drip method	115
Brewed by percolator	80
Instant	65
Tea	
Brewed (5-ounce cup)	40
Instant (5-ounce cup)	30
Iced (12-ounce cup)	70
Chocolate bar (6 ounces)	25
Soda pop	
Coca-Cola	46
Diet Coke	46
Pepsi-Cola	38
Diet Pepsi	36
Mountan Dew	54
Dr Pepper	40
Nonprescription drugs	
Dexatrim	200
No Doz	100
Vivarin	200
Excedrin	65
Triaminicin tablets	30
Dristan tablets	16

Figure 8–1

Caffeine Content of Selected Beverages, Foods, and Drugs

day each time the effects of the previous caffeine dose wear off.

Some people consume much more caffeine than they realize. An anthropology professor who suffered from insomnia estimated that he drank five cups of coffee a day. However, when he tallied his trips to the coffeepot, he found that his daily average was *nine* cups. Limiting his coffee consumption to the morning hours improved the quality of his sleep dramatically.

It is easy to measure how much you ingest by keeping track of the coffee, soda pop, and chocolate you take in each day. Use the table on page 140 to help you figure out the amount of caffeine in your diet.

As with alcohol, you can conduct a simple experiment to find out how caffeine consumption during the day affects your sleep. For a few days calculate the amount of caffeine you consume, and each day note the time when you take your last dose. Then, for each day, correlate the quality of your nighttime sleep with the amount of caffeine you had and when you had it.

Some people improve their sleep by limiting their caffeine intake to the morning hours. This strategy can be effective because the peak of caffeine's stimulating action is reached two to four hours after ingestion. However, because caffeine's stimulating effects can continue for up to twenty hours, some people must eliminate the drug entirely to improve their sleep.

If you decide to eliminate caffeine from your diet, it may not be easy for the first few days. As with any addictive drug, kicking a caffeine habit can cause withdrawal symptoms. When you stop consuming caffeine, you may lack energy or become sleepy during the day. You may be irritable, tense, or depressed. You may have headaches. Because of these drug-withdrawal reactions, it is better for many people to get off caffeine gradually rather than all at once.

Keep your goal in mind. If you give up caffeine or limit the amount you consume, you will almost certainly awaken more alert in the morning and sleep more soundly at night.

9

Depression

WE ALL FEEL SAD AT TIMES. BUT FOR SOME INDIVIDUALS these feelings are overwhelming and persist for long periods. Symptoms of depression vary from person to person. People who are depressed may lose interest in events and people around them. They may have difficulty thinking, concentrating, and remembering. They may feel apathetic and lethargic and lack motivation for performing routine daily activities. They often awaken in the predawn hours, unable to return to sleep.

About 20 percent of women and 10 percent of men experience an episode of serious depression at some time during their lives. During their lifetimes about 6 percent of women and 3 percent of men are hospitalized for depression.

Depression is not an all-or-nothing experience. At any given time, about one in five adults is experiencing some depressive symptoms.

ARE YOU DEPRESSED?

Before we go further, let's look at a checklist to measure whether and to what extent you experience depression. You can use this self-test to determine if you need to read this chapter. If the checklist indicates that you experience moderate or severe depression, read this chapter closely. But if the measure shows that you experience minimal or mild depression, you can skip ahead to the next chapter.

DEPRESSION AND SLEEP

Countless widows and widowers have lain awake in bed or paced the floor all night, too bereaved to sleep in spite of their exhaustion. Nearly all of us have lost sleep because we have been sad about some event, usually something much less disturbing than the loss of a spouse. In most cases our sleep returns to normal when the problem is resolved or when we begin to cope with it.

But people with serious depression experience poor sleep even when a problem is not weighing on their mind. In one out of five cases depression is accompanied by excessive sleep. This hypersomnia tends to accompany bipolar manic-depressive disorders.

Depressed people without manic episodes usually sleep less than before they became depressed. Often they fall asleep easily enough, only to awaken frequently during the night. They experience long and intensive REM sleep early in the night, and their deep, restorative sleep is reduced.

The most common depression-related sleep problem is awakening in the predawn hours with an inability to return to sleep at all. Chapter 11 will show us how a relatively new treatment, light therapy, can lessen this problem of early-morning awakening.

With many people there is a "chicken-versus-egg" question of whether depression causes their insomnia or in-

THE BURNS DEPRESSION CHECKLIST*

Instructions: The following is a list of symptoms that people sometimes have. Put a check (√) in the space to the right that best describes how much that symptom or problem has bothered you during the past week.

	0-NOT AT ALL	1-SOMEWHAT	2-MODERATELY	3-A LOT
1. **Sadness:** Have you been feeling sad or down in the dumps?				
2. **Discouragement:** Does the future look hopeless?				
3. **Low self-esteem:** Do you feel worthless or think of yourself as a failure?				
4. **Inferiority:** Do you feel inadequate or inferior to others?				
5. **Guilt:** Do you get self-critical and blame yourself for everything?				
6. **Indecivesness:** Do you have trouble making up your mind about things?				
7. **Irritability and frustration:** Have you been feeling resentful and angry a good deal of the time?				
8. **Loss of interest in life:** Have you lost interest in your career, your hobbies, your family, or your friends?				
9. **Loss of motivation:** Do you feel overwhelmed and have to push yourself hard to do things?				
10. **Poor self-image:** Do you think you're looking old or unattractive?				

(continued)

	0-NOT AT ALL	1-SOMEWHAT	2-MODERATELY	3-A LOT
11. **Appetite changes**: Have you lost your appetite? Or do you overeat or binge compulsively?				
12. **Sleep changes:** Do you suffer from insomnia and find it hard to get a good night's sleep? Or are you excessively tired and sleeping too much?				
13. **Loss of libido:** Have you lost your interest in sex?				
14. **Hypochondriasis:** Do you worry a great deal about your health?				
15. **Suicidal impulses†:** Do you have thoughts that life is not worth living or think that you might be better off dead?				

Add up your total score for the 15 symptoms and record it here: _____

Date: _____

†Anyone with suicidal urges should seek immediate consultation with a qualified psychiatrist or psychologist.

After you have completed the test, add up your total score. Give yourself one point for each item you checked "somewhat," two points for each item you checked "moderately," and three points for each item you checked "a lot." Your score will be somewhere between 0 (if you answered "not at all" for each of the 15 categories) and 45 (if you answered "a lot" for each one). Use this key to interpret your score.

Total score	Degree of Depression
0-4	Minimal or no depression
5-10	Borderline depression
11-20	Mild depression
21-30	Moderate depression
31-45	Severe depression

somnia causes their depression. In the book *Behavioral Treatment for Persistent Insomnia* (Pergamon Press, 1987), psychologist Patricia Lacks writes: "Sleep disturbance over some length of time appears to decrease a person's sense of general competence or confidence in the ability to handle problems. This negative self-attitude may then help to usher in feelings of depression that only exacerbate the sleep problem and lead to a downward spiral of lessening sleep and lowering mood."

Regardless of the origin of a depression-and-insomnia problem, the successful treatment of insomnia will improve depression, and the successful treatment of depression will improve insomnia. Part IV details procedures that reduce insomnia in nearly all instances. The remainder of this chapter discusses depression and ways to reduce its severity.

CAUSES OF DEPRESSION

Depression usually arises from a combination of factors, including genetic predisposition, negative events, and distorted thinking.

GENETIC PREDISPOSITION

Depression tends to run in families. Research examining the prevalence of depression among relatives has suggested that genetic factors contribute to depressive disorders. Some people are more vulnerable to becoming depressed.

The parents, siblings, and children of depressed people have a much greater risk of contracting depression than do more distant relatives. People with no depressed relatives are at lowest risk for depression. These findings hold true even when family members have been reared in different households.

Research with identical twins provides even stronger evidence that a predisposition to depression is genetically transmitted. Identical twins share identical genes. If one identical twin is depressed, there is a 70 percent probability that the other twin will also develop depression even when the twins are reared separately. This is striking evidence of a genetic predisposition to depression.

However, if genetic causes were the *only* risk factor, an identical twin would *invariably* develop depression when the other twin does. Because this does not happen, environmental factors such as unpleasant events are thought to contribute to depression. In some cases, life circumstances may determine whether a person becomes depressed, when it occurs, and for how long it lasts.

People who may be genetically predisposed to depression need not accept depression as their fate. There is much we can do to prevent depression and minimize its severity.

NEGATIVE EVENTS

Depression sometimes follows such life circumstances as loss of a job, financial reversal, retirement, serious medical illness, separation from friends, or the death of a loved one. However, in most cases there is no identifiable negative event that leads to depression. And most people who experience significant negative events do not consequently develop depression. It appears that a genetic predisposition is required for serious depression to develop in any particular individual.

DISTORTED THINKING

Two thousand years ago the Stoic philosophers of Greece and Rome developed the concept that what we think can make us feel bad. Epictetus wrote, "Men are disturbed not by things, but by the views they take of them." Similarly, Marcus Aurelius wrote, "If you are pained by any external thing, it is not this thing that disturbs you, but your own judgment about it. And it is in your power to wipe out this judgment now." Centuries later Shakespeare expressed the same idea in *Hamlet:* "There is nothing either good or bad, but thinking makes it so."

This ancient idea — that negative thoughts can trigger emotional distress — has been applied by some mental health professionals in understanding and treating depression. Psychiatrist David Burns states an extreme form of this viewpoint when writing about depression in his popular self-help book *Feeling Good:* "Every bad feeling you have is the result of your distorted negative thinking. Illogical pessimistic attitudes play the central role in the development and continuation of all your symptoms . . . the negative thoughts that flood your mind are the actual *cause* of your self-defeating emotions. These thoughts are what keep you lethargic and make you feel inadequate."

As an example of distorted thinking as an element of depression, consider these alternative ways to react to the death of a spouse. In a reaction of normal sadness a person would think, "I will miss the love and companionship we shared." But in the distorted thinking of depression, a person would have thoughts laden with negativity or self-blame:

- *"Life won't be worth living without him."*

- *"I'll never be happy again."*

- *"It's unfair that she died."*

- *"I should have done something to keep him from dying."*

There is evidence that depressed individuals do indeed perceive and describe their world in unrealistically negative ways. However, it may be that distorted thinking is simply a consequence of depression rather than its cause. Regardless of whether negative thoughts and perceptions cause or merely accompany depression, treatment that focuses on changing the negative thoughts of depression has proved very successful. This chapter later examines ways to identify and change the self-defeating thoughts of depression.

WHAT TO DO ABOUT DEPRESSION

Many people have used self-help techniques successfully to reduce their feelings of depression. Others have benefited from the more intensive and directive intervention of a counselor or psychotherapist. Still others require counseling or psychotherapy in combination with antidepressant medication. Let's look at these different ways of overcoming depression.

SELF-HELP TREATMENT

Behavioral Techniques

People with depression tend to be inactive, to stay home, and to avoid interacting with others. This may feel like the thing to do if you are depressed, because you lack the desire and energy to get out and do things. But if you follow your inclination to stay home all the time, you will remain depressed. Don't make the mistake of thinking that you will become more active after you get over your depression. The connection works in the opposite direction: You will get over your depression after you become more active.

The behavioral techniques below do not require any great skill to accomplish. All you have to do is to make the decision to get up and do them.

If you don't feel like it, fake it at first. Just go through the motions. Little by little, you will find that making a systematic effort to become more active will make you feel better. There are at least two ways you can do it.

Schedule Pleasant Activities

Many people with depression stop doing the things they used to enjoy. As a result, they feel that the fun has gone out of life. The relationship between depression and reduced pleasant activities is two-way. Doing few pleasant activities causes us to feel depressed, and feeling depressed causes us to do even fewer pleasant activities. The way to interrupt this cycle is to plan pleasant activities as part of your daily schedule.

Think of things you enjoyed doing when you felt happier. Then schedule some of these things every day. If you have difficulty thinking of pleasant activities you used to do, try some new things.

Three types of activities are particularly important in overcoming depression: (1) pleasant activities with other people we are fond of; (2) activities that make us feel useful and competent, such as making something or learning something new; (3) intrinsically pleasant activities, such as laughing, that are incompatible with being depressed.

If you have difficulty thinking of anything pleasant to do, here are some activities to choose from:

- *Get out of the city to enjoy nature.*
- *Look at the stars or moon.*
- *Go to a concert, lecture, movie, party, or sports event.*
- *See or smell flowers or plants.*
- *Buy something for yourself or someone else.*
- *Get new glasses.*
- *Have your hair cut.*
- *Play cards.*

- *Play a sport.*

- *Rent a comedy video. (For example, in* Anatomy of an Illness, *Norman Cousins documents the healing value of laughing at Marx Brothers films in his hospital bed.)*

- *Rent an absorbing drama video.*

- *Read a good book or magazine.*

- *Read a* Far Side *cartoon book.*

- *Plan a vacation.*

- *Eat good food.*

- *Walk your dog.*

- *Adopt a pet.*

- *Visit the zoo.*

- *Listen to music.*

- *Sing alone or in a group.*

- *Play a musical instrument.*

- *Do garden or yard work.*

- *Visit friends, or invite them over.*

- *Visit your parents, children, or other family members. (When turning to the company of others, don't talk about what's getting you down unless your companions can offer some specific help. Instead focus on activities to distract you from your troubles.)*

Whatever pleasant activities you choose, make sure that you develop a plan for when and how you will do them. If you have a regular job, schedule them for your hours after work and your days off. If you are retired or out of work, make a schedule for yourself all day. Try to do one or two pleasant things daily. When the time comes, resolve to do the scheduled activity even if you don't feel like it.

Physical Exercise

Exercise improves your state of mind. Aerobic exercise produces *endorphins*, chemicals in the brain related to the opiates that enhance one's sense of well-being. Hard exercise has been shown to elevate mood, increase the sense of control, and reduce feelings of depression.

In addition, exercise improves sleep in two important ways: It helps you fall asleep more easily, and it deepens your sleep. Exercise improves your sleep because of physiological changes that occur after you finish. Your body temperature rises about two degrees Fahrenheit while you are exercising hard. Subsequently, four to six hours later your body temperature drops to a level lower than it would be if you hadn't exercised at all. Because of this time lag before the rebound effect occurs, it is best to exercise about five hours before bedtime — in the late afternoon or early evening. But don't exercise close to bedtime, or your elevated body temperature will make it harder for you to fall asleep.

You don't have to exercise every day to reduce depression and improve sleep. What is most important is to achieve a state of cardiovascular fitness, and you can be fit if you exercise four times a week.

Warm up gradually for about five minutes. Then exercise hard enough to raise your heart rate, and keep moving briskly for twenty to thirty minutes. Finally, cool down gradually for another five or ten minutes, so you don't go directly from hard exercise to rest.

During your twenty to thirty minutes of sustained vigorous exercise, make sure that your heart rate reaches the aerobic target zone. (An aerobic exercise is one that improves heart and lung functioning by increasing oxygen consumption.) The chart on page 154 shows aerobic target zones for different ages. Just find the age closest to yours;

Age	Target Zone, Beats per Minute
20	120 - 150
25	117 - 146
30	114 - 142
35	111 - 138
40	108 -135
45	105 - 131
50	102 - 127
55	99 - 123
60	96 - 120
65	93 - 116
70	90 - 113

Figure 9–2

then read across to find how fast your pulse should beat while you are exercising hard.

While you are exercising, pause and take your pulse to be sure it is in your target zone. To measure your heart rate, count your wrist pulse for fifteen seconds and multiply by four. If your heart rate is beneath your target zone, you need to exercise more vigorously.

Some people have a hard time finding their pulse, or feel it is too complicated to calculate their heart rate. For a simple alternative, they can just exercise hard enough to breathe heavily.

You might be wondering what kind of exercise you should do. It's your choice. Just be sure that it makes you work enough to get your heart rate up and to get you breathing hard. Walking is a good activity for people who don't like to do formal exercise. Many people exercise by walking briskly, with their arms swinging up and down to increase exertion. You can also carry small weights designed to work out your upper body as you walk. Jogging intermittently for a few seconds now and then interspersed with walking will boost your heart rate.

Other activities include running, dancing, swimming, bicycling, playing tennis, or doing aerobic workouts in a class or with a video. Consider putting an exercise bike or rowing machine in front of your TV so you can work out while watching the evening news or a videotaped program. Choose an exercise you enjoy — or used to enjoy — because you will be more likely to keep up an enjoyable exercise.

You may feel that you are too depressed and don't have enough energy to exercise, especially if you haven't been sleeping well at night. But try anyway. If you exercise regularly, you will find that during the day and evening you have more energy, because exercise actually counteracts fatigue. Not only that, but *you will sleep better at night.*

Cognitive Techniques

Earlier in the chapter we saw how the things we tell ourselves can contribute to depression. A very effective movement in mental health — *cognitive therapy* — uses positive thoughts to counteract the negative thoughts of depression.

The word "cognitive" comes from "cognition," which means thought or perception. In 1955 psychologist Albert Ellis originated cognitive therapy, which is based on the assumption that the things we tell ourselves — or *self-talk* — can make us feel either depressed or happy. Cognitive therapy can be utilized with a professional therapist or in a self-help mode.

A study conducted throughout the 1980s at the National Institute of Mental Health found short-term cognitive therapy as effective as drug treatment with the antidepressant imipramine for mild and moderate depression.

Depression-prone people tend to have unrealistically negative attitudes about themselves, their environments, and their futures. Let's examine some negative, distorted thoughts that can lead to or aggravate depression. After each depressive thought, look at the alternative, more positive thought you can substitute in the same situation.

NEGATIVE SELF-TALK	POSITIVE ALTERNATIVES
"My future is bleak."	"I'll write down what steps I can take to improve my future."
"I'm just not cut out to do sales."	"She wasn't really interested in our selection."
"What's the use?"	"It's worth a try."
"I'm a failure."	"I failed the biology test, but there's time to bring my grade up. And I'm doing well in my other subjects."
"I'm a lousy parent."	"I lost my temper and yelled at the kids, but that was just one time."
"What's wrong with me?"	"I've been feeling depressed, but I'm working to get better."
"I look like shit."	"I'll look better and feel better if I wash my hair and put on clean clothes."
"Why bother getting up?"	"Even though I don't feel like it, I'll plan something fun today."

The way to change negative thoughts is to identify their presence, dispute their faulty logic, and substitute more positive self-talk. Every time you find yourself feeling depressed, try to find negative thoughts like the ones on the left, in the table above, and substitute more positive thoughts like the ones on the right. If you regularly make the effort to change the way you think, you will change the way you *feel*.

Recommended Self-Help Resources

There are many self-help books available for dealing with depression. These are among the best:

- David Burns, *Feeling Good* (New York: Morrow, 1980). This is a clear and comprehensive presentation of the principles of cognitive therapy as a treatment for depression.

- Peter Lewinsohn and others, *Control Your Depression* (Englewood Cliffs, N.J.: Prentice-Hall, 1986). This describes a program that includes cognitive therapy and behavioral approaches for treating depression.

- Albert Ellis and Robert Harper, *A New Guide to Rational Living* (Englewood Cliffs, N.J.: Prentice-Hall, 1975). This classic self-help book shows how to use cognitive methods to overcome depression and other emotional disorders.

WHEN AND HOW TO FIND PROFESSIONAL HELP

If you experience mild or moderate levels of depression, try the self-help resources described in this chapter. If you need additional help, or if you suffer more severe depression, it is best to work with a mental health specialist — a psychiatrist, psychologist, social worker, counselor, or psychiatric nurse.

Antidepressant medications have proved very helpful in treating moderate and severe depression. If you are open to the idea of antidepressant medication, make sure that the specialist you choose either is a psychiatrist or can work closely with your doctor or another physician who will consider prescribing medication.

There are several ways to find a qualified mental health specialist:

- *Ask your doctor.*

- *Call your state mental health licensing board.*

- *Call your state's chapter of the American Psychiatric Association or the American Psychological Association. You can get the numbers of your local chapters from the national offices in Washington, D.C., at 202-682-6220 or 202-336-5700 respectively.*

- *Call the department of psychiatry, psychology, social work, or counseling at a nearby university.*

Be a careful consumer. When you speak with the referring person or inquire by phone at the mental health specialist's office, be sure to ask about the specialist's background and experience in using cognitive and behavioral techniques for treating depression. Even if you take antidepressant drugs, it is best to learn and use these proven antidepression methods. If the counselor or therapist uses another approach, keep inquiring until you find someone who has experience with cognitive and behavioral techniques for treating depression.

10
Stress and Anxiety

STRESS AND ANXIETY CAN CAUSE DIFFICULTY FALLING asleep, frequent awakenings during the night, lighter sleep, or early-morning awakening. This chapter includes diagnostic inventories to help you estimate how much stress and anxiety you experience and to determine how closely you need to read the subjects in this chapter:

- *The interrelated and overlapping concepts of stress and anxiety*
- *What to do about the stress response of anger*
- *How stress and anxiety can contribute to insomnia*
- *Ways to manage day-to-day stress and anxiety*
- *What to do about different anxiety disorders that are more severe than everyday anxiety*

A STRESS INVENTORY

The stress inventory below includes the kinds of irritants, pressures, and problems that often cause stress. Put a check by each stressor that has bothered you significantly during the past week.

FAMILY STRESSORS

___ 1. Concern about your relationship with your spouse or significant other
___ 2. Concern about your children (their health, behavior, friends, etc.)
___ 3. Concern about other family members

JOB STRESSORS

___ 4. Dissatisfaction with the kind of work you do
___ 5. Concern about your job performance generally or on a specific project
___ 6. Concern about job security
___ 7. Problems with your boss
___ 8. Problems with co-workers
___ 9. Problems with clients or customers

FINANCIAL STRESSORS

___ 10. Not enough money for basic necessities
___ 11. Concern about long-term financial security

HEALTH STRESSORS

___ 12. Concern about not getting enough rest or sleep
___ 13. Concern about habits such as caffeine, tobacco, or alcohol
___ 14. Other concerns about your health

OTHER STRESSORS

___ 15. Problems with a person or group other than your family, boss, or co-workers
___ 16. Too many things to do or not enough time to get things done
___ 17. Household chores (cleaning, errands, home or car maintenance)
___ 18. Losing or breaking an important item
___ 19. Commuting to work
___ 20. Concern about crime

Stress from even one stressor can disrupt sleep. The more items you checked, the more you can benefit from learning and practicing the stress-management techniques in this chapter.

STRESS

The word "stress" is often considered a synonym for anything outside us that is troubling or unpleasant. Among experts, however, stress is considered *the state of arousal with which the body meets perceived threats or challenges.*

A stressor is a stimulus that leads to the stress response. Stressors consist of the challenges and threats we perceive in our environment, as well as the things we tell ourselves about stressors. An example of a challenge is the prospect of making an important presentation. An example of a perceived threat is someone questioning your competence. An example of what we tell ourselves about a stressor is the thought "I can't take any more of these hassles."

The stress response evolved to help us survive as individuals and as a species. Let's see how stress was adaptive to survival in prehistoric times and why it no longer is such a good thing.

Imagine that it is a prehistoric day when our ancestors

were evolving. You are a protohuman *Homo habilis* two million years ago, or a *Homo erectus* half a million years ago, or a *Homo sapiens* fifty thousand years ago. As you quietly dig for roots and insects to eat, you see a movement at the edge of your vision. A predatory animal — a saber-toothed tiger, cave bear, or dire wolf — is moving toward you, its head down as it follows your scent. You know that you have only two choices if you are to survive: You can defend yourself or you can flee.

Faced with this "fight or flight" demand, your body reacts instantly in many ways:

- *Adrenaline is released into your bloodstream, overcoming any effects of fatigue.*

- *Your breathing becomes more shallow as it speeds up to supply increased oxygen to your muscles.*

- *Your heart rate and blood pressure increase, as blood rushes from your hands and feet to the large muscles of your arms and legs.*

- *Blood-clotting mechanisms are activated, so less blood will be lost in case of injury.*

- *Perspiration cools your body, allowing it to burn more energy.*

- *Your muscles tense to prepare for action.*

- *Sugars and fats from your liver flood your body with fuel for quick energy.*

- *Saliva dries up and digestion stops, so that blood can be diverted to the muscles and brain.*

The stress response was adaptive for prehistoric humans throughout evolution: It enabled them to fight or flee quickly in response to very real dangers in their environment. As modern humans, we retain the automatic stress response that helped our ancestors survive. Today, though, our bodies prepare us for fights or flights that never occur.

Although the stressors that aroused early humans have largely disappeared, the primitive stress response remains unchanged. The stress response that prepares us for business meetings is identical to that which prepared our ancestors for physical confrontations. But instead of fierce animals and hostile tribes, we deal with bosses, office politics, deadlines, snarled traffic, money problems, and the behavior of our kids.

In contrast to our prehistoric progenitors, today we have few outlets for our stress response and few physical demands to release the energy it produces. Instead we turn the energy inward, and this can lead to physical and emotional problems. But as we will see, there are ways to contain our stress response or to vent the energy it creates in our bodies.

WHAT'S BAD ABOUT STRESS

Not only does the stress response fail to prepare us for modern stressors, but it can lead to distress and to stress-related illnesses. For example, the physiological response of blood clotting during stress was adaptive in prehistoric times, because it reduced bleeding in a physical confrontation. But the same blood-clotting mechanism today is more likely to lead to a heart attack or stroke. Similarly, digestive changes during the stress response that direct the blood away from the stomach can lead to ulcers.

The office of the United States surgeon general has declared that excessive stress can have serious implications for the physical and mental health of Americans. Stress contributes to many types of diseases:

- *Gastrointestinal disorders, such as ulcers and heartburn*
- *Cardiovascular disorders, such as hypertension and migraine headaches*
- *Respiratory disorders, such as asthma and allergies*
- *Musculoskeletal disorders, such as arthritis and low back pain*
- *Inhibition of the immune system*

Stress affects not only our bodies but also the ways we think and feel. Stress can contribute to anxiety disorders and depression. Think about the times when you came home feeling tense and irritable after a particularly bad day at work or when you felt agitated after an argument with someone close to you.

We can bounce back from occasional stress at work or in other situations. But if stress continues unabated day after day, we are likely to feel helpless, hopeless, depressed, or anxious.

Stress contributes directly to insomnia. Research shows that people get less deep, restorative sleep on nights when they are experiencing stress. Trouble falling asleep and trouble staying asleep are common during stressful periods.

THE GOOD NEWS ABOUT STRESS

Not all stress is harmful. Lower levels of stress help us be productive. Our "fight or flight" stress response provides us with energy for getting things done and with much of our zest and excitement for living. In fact, we even are willing to pay to experience stress: We gamble, watch action movies, and ride roller coasters. Hans Selye, the foremost pioneer of stress research, writes in *Stress Without Distress* (New York: Lippincott, 1980): "Stress is the spice of life. . . .

Who would enjoy a life of no runs, no hits, no errors?"

Stress gives us that extra push to complete a big project or to keep up with a multitude of small ones. If we experience very low levels of stress, we have difficulty performing efficiently or being productive. As stress rises, our productivity increases — to a point. We reach the level of peak performance when stress mobilizes us enough to achieve what we have to do. When we begin to experience too much stress, we may feel overloaded and overwhelmed. Performance and productivity then decline.

Our goal, then, is not to relieve ourselves of all our stress, or even most of it. Instead our goal is to learn two skills: to recognize when we are experiencing too much stress and to manage unnecessary stress that interferes with our productivity and well-being.

WHERE STRESS COMES FROM

Much popular writing theorizes that stress derives from highly significant life events, such as the loss of your job or the death of a close friend. However, research that is more recent and better designed shows that most stress comes not from large-scale events but rather from small day-to-day hassles.

Our everyday stress comes from many different sources. The clearest way to think about stressors is to consider them in two categories: stressors imposed from *outside* (your situation) and stressors generated from *inside* (your thoughts).

Stress from Situations

Stressors come from many external sources, ranging from social interaction to unpleasant working conditions. A stressor can be anything that you perceive as a threat or a challenge.

Family stressors come in many forms. The birth of a child places new demands on the other family members. Sibling rivalry and quarrels raise the physical arousal of everyone in the household. A teenager's desire to become independent conflicts with the parents' responsibility for supervision.

In the past, a typical family was a resilient structure that provided support and helped everyone in it to cope with outside stressors. Today, however, nearly half of all marriages end in divorce, and the changes that result from divorce supply new sources of stress to parents and children.

Job stressors include bosses, cramped offices, difficult co-workers, demanding clients, project deadlines, and dislike of the kind of work you do. A government task force study on longevity found that, after tobacco use and genetic inheritance, job satisfaction is the most accurate predictor of longevity.

People stressors are found in our families and workplaces, as we saw above. They also include such people as noisy neighbors and rude store clerks. People stressors vary greatly from person to person. Some of us enjoy the challenge of asking someone for a date, attending a party, or giving a speech. Others find such interactions with people stressful.

Financial stressors are bills, mortgages, money shortages, and concerns about long-term financial security.

Health stressors include chemical stressors — substances we ingest such as caffeine and nicotine, that can cause stress responses. Other stressors are concerns about health, weight, and health-related habits.

Change stressors can occur whenever we alter any routine important in our lives. We may experience stress when we leave a job and begin a new one, when we move to a new neighborhood, when we marry, or when we retire.

Other stressors in our lives include commuting, weather extremes, upsetting local or national events, and irritants like losing or breaking an important item.

Stress from Your Thoughts

It is commonly thought that all stress comes from other people and problems around us. However, much of our stress comes not from sources external to ourselves but from our thoughts.

In the previous chapter, we saw how irrational beliefs and distorted thinking can contribute to depression. Similarly, negative thoughts can aggravate stress, anxiety, and anger. Later in this chapter techniques are presented for identifying and changing irrational beliefs and distorted thinking that contribute to anxiety and stress.

ANGER AS A STRESS RESPONSE

Many people suffer insomnia as a result of anger about something that happened during the day. They lie awake in bed, mulling over a conflict or wishing they had thought of something else to do or say in a confrontation.

Anger is an emotional stress response in which we prepare ourselves for a fight rather than for flight. Like other stress responses, anger is accompanied by heightened physiological arousal, and it begins from external stressors and increases in intensity as the result of negative self-talk.

Anger can be controlled by the stress-management methods detailed later in this chapter. They can help you reduce the effects of anger so that it doesn't interfere with your sleep.

ANXIETY

We all feel anxious at times, when something close to us is threatened or when we are awaiting an unpleasant confrontation. In fact, the experience of anxiety is often considered a mark of our humanness. Our period in history was called the "Age of Anxiety" by the poet W. H. Auden. But just what is anxiety? It is a feeling of fear or apprehension that is accompanied by such signs of physiological arousal as a rapid heartbeat, fast and shallow breathing, and muscle tension.

There is substantial overlap between the concepts of stress and anxiety. A stress response and an anxiety response each involve heightened physiological activity. Each may be developed by our thoughts and attitudes. But there is one major difference between stress and anxiety: Stress always involves an external stressor. Although people's stress responses are often heightened by what they tell themselves, with stress there is an emphasis on environmental events that initiated the response. In contrast, anxiety may be experienced without any apparent external stressor that precipitated the feeling. *It can come from inside you.*

AN ANXIETY INVENTORY

The stress inventory focused on your reaction to external events as causes of stress. In contrast, this anxiety inventory focuses on the internal feelings, thoughts, and physiological events that constitute the experience of anxiety. Put a check in the space to the left of each symptom that has bothered you significantly during the past week.

THOUGHTS AND FEELINGS

___ 1. Apprehension, worry, or fear, either in response to a specific situation or for no apparent reason

___ 2. Sudden unexpected panic spells

___ 3. A feeling that you're on the verge of losing control

___ 4. Fears about looking foolish or inadequate in front of others

___ 5. Fears of being alone, isolated, or abandoned

___ 6. Fears of objects or situations

___ 7. Recurrent persistent thoughts that intrude upon your mind (e.g., the thought that you have hurt someone or that your hands are contaminated)

___ 8. Compulsions to repeat behaviors to an irrational degree (e.g., repeatedly washing your hands or checking that a door is locked)

PHYSICAL RESPONSES NOT BROUGHT ON BY EXERCISE

___ 9. Racing or pounding of the heart

___ 10. Tight, tense muscles

___ 11. A lump in the throat

___ 12. Cold or sweaty hands

___ 13. Trembling or shaking

___ 14. Feeling generally nervous or on edge

If you answered yes to none of the items, you don't have a current problem with anxiety. But if you answered yes to *any* item, your insomnia may be due to excessive anxiety or an anxiety disorder, and you can benefit from reading the rest of this chapter.

ANXIETY AND THE ANXIETY DISORDERS

Anxiety appears at different levels of intensity and in different forms. Its severity ranges from the fleeting feeling of uneasiness to the debilitating terror of a panic attack.

Anxiety can be a normal reaction to threatening situations, such as danger and medical illness. Approximately one-third of the adult population experiences significant feelings of anxiety. However, about 3 percent of adults experience anxiety of such intensity and long duration that it is considered an anxiety disorder. If the anxiety was triggered by a particular event, it may persist for months instead of dissipating after the triggering event has gone away.

Like most mental disorders, anxiety disorders are inherited to a large degree. This doesn't mean that people predictably inherit specific types of anxiety disorders from their parents. Instead, people tend to inherit general personality types that predispose them to be overly anxious. In addition, certain childhood circumstances may lead people to anxious ways of perceiving the world and behaving.

Let's review the seven major types of anxiety disorders. These categories are not mutually exclusive, and one person can experience symptoms from more than one category.

Generalized Anxiety Disorder

This disorder is characterized by chronic anxiety and worry that lasts for at least six months. Typically it first appears in a person's twenties or thirties, and it is equally common in men and women.

Behavioral treatments for generalized anxiety disorder include relaxation, exercise, and adopting thoughts and self-talk that promote a calmer and more accepting attitude toward life. We will explore each of these in the last section of this chapter.

Panic Disorder

A panic disorder manifests itself in panic attacks — sudden episodes of extreme apprehension or fear that occur with no apparent cause. A panic disorder usually first appears in a person's twenties, although it can also develop later in life.

Panic disorder is the anxiety disorder for which medication is prescribed most often. The drug chosen is usually the antianxiety agent Xanax — a benzodiazepine, in the same drug family as the most commonly prescribed sleeping pills. The antidepressant Tofranil is sometimes effective as well.

Like generalized anxiety disorder, panic disorder can be treated through relaxation, exercise, and methods of adopting calmer thoughts and self-talk.

Agoraphobia

The word "agoraphobia" means "fear of the marketplace." This disorder is a fear of being caught in a place from which escape might be difficult or where help might be unavailable in case of sudden incapacitation such as from a panic attack. Agoraphobics fear being in public places because they cannot easily escape. Ordinary activities, such as driving or grocery shopping, may be difficult or impossible, and the person may become housebound.

Agoraphobia tends to appear in the late teens or early twenties. The disorder is more prevalent among women than men.

The most effective treatment for agoraphobia is identical to the treatment of choice for *all* phobias: The individual must face the feared object or situation. Sufficient exposure to the feared situation will cause the fear to diminish and eventually to disappear. People who persist in confronting the feared situation find out that there are no realistic terrible consequences after all.

Exposure can also be done in fantasy, by imagining the feared situation vividly. Gradual exposure to the feared situation is called *desensitization*. In desensitization, the person begins with imagined exposure to a situation that is just slightly frightening, then step by step confronts situations that are more feared.

Social Phobia

People with this disorder irrationally fear embarrassment in situations in which they are exposed to the scrutiny of others. People with social phobias tend to avoid being with other people. In most cases, social phobia first appears in late childhood or early adolescence.

Like agoraphobia, social phobia is best treated by facing the feared situation.

Simple Phobia

Simple phobia involves an irrational fear and avoidance of one type of object or situation. By definition, the class of simple phobias excludes agoraphobia and social phobias. Simple phobias affect about one in ten men and one in five women at some time in their lives. Among the most common simple phobias are fears of animals, close spaces, and heights.

The most effective treatment for simple phobias is the same as that for agoraphobia and social phobia described above.

Obsessive Compulsive Disorder

There are two features of this disorder. *Obsessions* are recurrent thoughts or impulses that feel senseless or repugnant and that intrude persistently into one's mind. The most common obsessions involve contamination, violence, or doubt. *Compulsions* are repetitive irrational behaviors — such as checking a light switch or washing one's hands — that usually are performed to dispel the anxiety caused by obsessions.

Obsessive compulsive disorder is treated by the behavioral strategy of *exposure and response prevention*. This treatment involves exposing the person to situations that arouse obsessions and compulsions, then preventing him or her from engaging in those obsessive thoughts or compulsive behaviors. This causes anxiety to increase initially, then to decrease markedly.

Many people with this disorder find that obsessions and compulsions decrease when they are treated with the antidepressants clomipramine (Anafranil) or fluoxetine (Prozac).

Whether or not the person responds to medication, he or she needs to learn behavioral learning principles to minimize obsessive and compulsive behaviors. The best treatment for obsessive compulsive disorder is a combination of medication and behavior therapy.

The Obsessive Compulsive Foundation publishes a newsletter and other literature. It provides information on behavior therapists experienced in working with the disorder as well as support groups in different areas. You can contact this organization at 9 Depot Street, Milford, CT 06460; 203-878-5669.

Post-Traumatic Stress Disorder

People with this disorder develop anxious symptoms following a traumatic event, such as a natural disaster or car accident. Symptoms may appear immediately or soon after the trauma, or they may not emerge until months or even years later.

Post-traumatic stress disorder can be alleviated by relaxation, exercise, and adoption of calming self-talk. In addition, counseling can help the person work through such feelings as fear, loss, or guilt that may surround the original traumatic event.

LEARN TO MANAGE YOUR STRESS AND ANXIETY

We saw earlier that the benzodiazepine (BZD) medications are sometimes prescribed to treat anxiety disorders. A good guideline is to use medication only if anxiety is disrupting your life significantly. If you consider taking medication for an anxiety problem, be sure to discuss with your physician any side effects, interactions with alcohol and other drugs, the likelihood of dependence, and the projected duration of medication treatment.

The BZD Xanax is often prescribed to treat anxiety. Xanax is the fifth most frequently prescribed drug in the United States. As with any BZD, regular use for more than a few weeks can lead to problems with tolerance and withdrawal.

In this section we will consider stress management and anxiety management jointly, for two reasons. First, there is considerable overlap between stress and anxiety responses. Second, there is much overlap between the methods for treating stress and those for treating anxiety reactions. In the rest of the chapter we will review the four most effective ways to manage stress and anxiety:

- *Reduce external stressors, such as insufficient time and difficult people in your life.*

- *Exercise.*

- *Learn relaxation methods.*

- *Learn ways to reduce internal stressors by changing the things you say to yourself.*

MANAGE EXTERNAL STRESSORS

One way to reduce everyday stress and anxiety is to learn skills for coping with your external stressors. For example, skills related to time management will help you reduce the severity of the common stressor of having insufficient time to get things done. Assertiveness skills and other communication skills can help you with another common stressor: dealing with difficult people.

Techniques for time management, assertiveness, and dealing with people are included in the stress-management books recommended at the end of this chapter.

EXERCISE AWAY YOUR STRESS AND ANXIETY

We saw in the previous chapter on depression that exercise produces endorphins — naturally occurring chemicals in the brain that lead to a sense of calm and well-being. We also saw that aerobic exercise can reduce the effects of depression. In a similar way, the beneficial effects of exercise can help you manage your everyday stress and anxiety.

The stress response is nature's way of preparing you for muscular exertion. In turn, energetic physical exercise is a natural way to utilize and vent the stress response once it has begun. During exercise, potentially harmful elements of the stress response — such as lactic acid, thyroxin, and adrenaline — are used in a healthful manner.

A second benefit of vigorous exercise is that it helps you learn more effectively the relaxation exercises presented in the section below. When you exercise regularly, your muscles become better toned — that is, they become more responsive and capable of performing work. And better muscle tone promotes more effective muscular relaxation.

To use exercise as a tool for managing your stress and anxiety, follow the exercise guidelines on pages 153–155. Being in a state of aerobic fitness helps you inoculate yourself not only from depression but also from the effects of stress and anxiety.

LEARN AND USE RELAXATION SKILLS

Remember that stress and anxiety are physical experiences as well as mental experiences. Maladaptive body changes during stress and anxiety responses include fast, shallow breathing, increased heart rate, and tense muscles.

There are two benefits of learning relaxation skills. First, by practicing physical relaxation during the day and evening, you will lower your general level of physical tension. Second, by learning to utilize physical relaxation on the spot, you can ease or eliminate tension when you find yourself in a particularly stressful or anxious situation.

Many insomnia sufferers experience heightened physiological arousal at bedtime. Chapter 15 reviews ways to use relaxation at bedtime to help induce sleep. But don't begin by practicing these exercises at bedtime. Use them at bedtime only after you have practiced them during the day and early evening and have acquired some skill at them.

Each of the following methods of relaxation has proved to reduce stress and anxiety in some people. Quickly review the techniques; then experiment with one or more of them. See which one or ones you feel most comfortable with. Then focus on that technique or techniques. These are the techniques we will cover:

- *Scanning for tension*

- *Abdominal breathing*

- *Meditation and yoga*

- *Tense-and-release relaxation*

- *Passive relaxation*

- *Autogenic relaxation*

- *Mental imagery*

- *Biofeedback*

In addition, we will examine problems a few people — one in thirty — have with relaxation. Finally, you will see how to choose a relaxation technique that works for you.

Scanning for Tension

The first step in using relaxation exercises is to find out how much tension is in your body and where it is stored.

Scanning for tension can be paired with any of several relaxation exercises.

You can check yourself for tension at bedtime or any time during the day or night. Scanning is like X-raying each part of your body and looking for tightness. Scanning gives you awareness of your tension. With practice, you will be able to scan your body in a few seconds. Here's how to do it.

1. Lie down or sit comfortably in a chair that supports your head. Uncross your arms and legs. Close your eyes if it helps you focus on your body.
2. In your mind's eye, begin to scan the sensations in your body, looking for tension or tightness. Start at the fingers of both hands. Slowly scan up through your forearms and upper arms.
3. Move your attention to the top of your head. Scan down through your forehead, the area around your eyes, and your jaw. Check to see if your teeth are clenched.
4. From your head, scan down to your neck, shoulder, back, and chest muscles. Look for tension or tightness in each muscle group.
5. Notice your breathing. Check to see if it is rapid and shallow, rather than slow and deep.
6. Focus your attention on your hips. Scan for tension. Then move slowly down your thighs and calves. Check your toes for curling or tightness.

Next we will see what you can do about the tension you find.

Abdominal Breathing

When you find muscle tension or fast and shallow breathing, the simplest way to restore relaxation is to change the way you are breathing. Voluntary control of breathing is the world's oldest stress and anxiety reduction technique, dating back thousands of years. Again, lie down or sit comfortably with your head supported, and close your eyes if you wish.

Breathe in slowly through your nose as you count to five in your mind: "In, one, two, three, four, five." Leave about one second between each number. First fill your stomach area with air, then your chest.

Your stomach and then your chest will rise as you inhale. You may not be comfortable with the feeling of your stomach rising. Extending your stomach contradicts what you have been told since childhood: to keep your stomach in. In abdominal breathing, however, an extended stomach simply means that you have inflated the lower lobes of your lungs with air.

When you reach the number five, your lungs will be nearly full. Hold in the air for three seconds; then slowly release it through your nose or mouth. Count backward in your mind this time: "Out, five, four, three, two, one." Be sure to empty your lungs.

Repeat the in-and-out breathing exercise two more times. Like scanning, this exercise takes about a half minute initially. When you put scanning and abdominal breathing together, you have a simple and effective one-minute technique to breathe away tension as soon as you find it. All you need is the time it takes to breathe in and out three times.

1. As you breathe in, scan your face, neck, shoulders, and arms. As you breathe out, let any tension in those areas slip away.
2. As you breathe in again, scan your chest and stomach. As you breathe out, let any tension in those areas slip away.
3. As you breathe in a third time, scan your hips, legs, and feet. As you breathe out, let any tension in those areas slip away.

Next we will look at two ancient forms of breath control that can be useful for reducing stress and anxiety.

Meditation and Yoga

Meditation is a method of inducing quiet inner reflection. Like deep breathing and other forms of relaxation, meditation decreases heart rate and muscle tension, leading to a reduced feeling of stress and anxiety. Meditation requires the person to concentrate on a repetitive stimulus while sitting quietly in a restful state.

All forms of meditation are intended to quiet the body and the mind. Transcendental meditation involves concentrating on a *mantra* — a calming word or phrase. Zen meditation requires concentrating on one's breathing. Other forms of meditation involve focusing on a lighted candle or some other stimulus.

The word *Yoga* means "union or oneness with life." Like meditation, yoga involves muscle relaxation and patterns of breathing. Yoga as an approach to stress management requires no acceptance of Hindu religious teachings.

Yoga and meditation methods must be learned from a trainer rather than a mental-health specialist. If you are interested in learning about these techniques, look in the yellow pages under "Meditation Instruction" or "Yoga Instruction." Or inquire at a YMCA, continuing education program, college, or university.

Now that we have examined different forms of the ancient practice of achieving relaxation through breath control, we will turn to more recent developments in techniques for reducing stress and anxiety.

Tense-and-Release Relaxation

When a muscle is tensed for a few seconds, it tends to become relaxed afterward even more than before the tensing. When you make use of this fact, tense-and-release relaxation can help you achieve a deeply relaxed state. Like other types of relaxation, this one should be done lying down or seated in a comfortable chair — preferably a recliner — with your head supported.

Detailed instructions are presented in Appendix 1. You may want to record your own relaxation tape, using the three kinds of relaxation instructions in that appendix.

Alternatively, you can learn relaxation from commercially available cassette recordings. Sources are listed later in this chapter.

Passive Relaxation

Passive relaxation is simpler and quicker to learn than the tense-and-release method. When using passive relaxation, you direct your attention to the same muscle groups as in the tense-and-release method. But you omit the part where you tense your muscles. Instead, you just gently let go of the tension in each muscle group when you reach it.

It is best to practice tense-and-release relaxation several times before trying passive relaxation. The tense-and-release method tends to induce deeper levels of relaxation than the passive method. If you learn the tense-and-release method first, you can recall the deep relaxation from that method and use it in passive relaxation. Passive relaxation is sometimes called *recall relaxation* for this reason.

Instructions for passive relaxation are presented in Appendix 1. As with the tense-and-release method, you can make your own relaxation tape or buy a commercial one.

Autogenic Relaxation

The word "autogenic" means "self-generating." Any form of self-guided relaxation may be considered autogenic. However, the term has come to refer specifically to methods of concentrating passively on verbal suggestions of relaxation and calm.

Like the previous two forms of relaxation, autogenic exercises can help you reverse the action of the body's stress response. During the "fight-or-flight" reaction, blood tends to pool in the trunk and head. Verbal suggestions such as "My right hand is warm" can help direct more blood to your hand, warming and relaxing it. Similarly, a suggestion like "My forehead is cool" can help reduce blood flow to the head. The suggestion "My heartbeat is calm" can help slow down heart rate.

Appendix 1 presents instructions for autogenic relaxation.

Mental Imagery

Mental imagery is the mind's most basic way of learning and storing information. Aristotle wrote, "The mind never thinks without a picture." Mental images include sights ("the mind's eye") as well as sound, smell, and touch.

The images in your mind affect how you feel and even how your body behaves physiologically. To create a relaxing image, choose a pleasant and restful scene you are familiar with. Imagine yourself resting in a meadow with grazing cows and horses; lying on the beach, feeling and smelling the warm salt air washing over your body; floating on a cloud in warm gentle air; lying in a snug sleeping bag as snowflakes drift all around you. Be sure to see the sights, hear the sounds, smell the scents, and feel the sensations.

Appendix 2 presents one example of mental imagery that you can use at bedtime or other times to help you relax.

Biofeedback

This is a method of learning to control such physiological functions as heart rate, blood pressure, muscle tension, and brain waves. By using biofeedback instruments, you can learn which mental states accompany different physiological changes. With this awareness, you can learn to influence your body's levels of tension and relaxation.

Research has shown that in most instances biofeedback is no more effective than other methods of relaxation.

What to Do When Thoughts or Images Intrude

Sometimes people attempting to relax have difficulty with intrusive thoughts or images. Don't be upset if you lose your concentration and find something other than relaxation in your mind. Several methods can be used to cope with interfering thoughts or images. Regardless of which one works best for you, it may be necessary to apply the technique and refocus several times before the intrusive thoughts or images disappear.

The first method of coping with this problem takes advantage of an interesting fact: Our subvocal speech muscles are often activated when verbal thoughts are in our mind, and the muscles around the eyes are activated when we experience visual images. Because of this mind-body connection, if you deeply relax the speech muscles — tongue, lips, jaws, throat, and cheeks — you will reduce the presence of undesired thoughts. So when you find intrusive thoughts, focus harder on relaxing your speech muscles. Similarly, for intrusive visual images, focus on relaxing the muscles around your eyes. This increased emphasis on relaxing the speech muscles or the eyes can be combined with the other kinds of techniques below.

A second method of coping with intrusive thoughts and images is thought stopping. As soon as a thought or image intrudes, shout the word "STOP!" You can shout it aloud, whisper it, or "shout" it in your mind. As simple as it seems, this technique often works. It eliminates the negative thought long enough for you to reorient yourself to your relaxation. After thought stopping, immediately refocus on your breathing and the feelings of relaxation.

A third method involves switching abruptly from the intrusive thought or image to a pleasant image or scene in your mind's eye.

A fourth method is to visualize getting rid of the distracting thought. Imagine the thought or image written in sand at the beach; then let the ocean's waves wash it away. Or imagine writing the thought or image on a piece of paper. Next imagine a balloon with a string. Roll up the paper with the thought or image on it, tie it to the balloon string, and let the balloon go. Watch it drift up into the sky. When it is nearly out of sight, refocus on your breathing and relaxation.

A fifth method is to use a mantra — a calming word or phrase. We noted earlier that using a mantra is an integral part of meditation. Focusing on a mantra can be helpful in reducing intrusive thoughts or images. You can choose any two-syllable word or phrase. Use the first syllable when you breathe in and the second when you breathe out. Mantras that work for some people are "Be calm," "Heavy," "Floating," and "At peace." Other people say the word "one" or the Sanskrit word "*om*," which means the same thing. Because many people find that the word "relax" paradoxically makes them tense, it is better to choose another mantra.

If you find that thoughts or images return so quickly that you can't concentrate on your relaxation, you may need to stop practicing and do something else. Sometimes it is best to take care of the concern you keep thinking about, then relax after you have finished with it.

A Caution About Relaxation

Paradoxically, 3 to 4 percent of people experience an anxiety response to relaxation methods. Instead of becoming calm and relaxed, they become tense and anxious. For some people this reaction comes from a feeling that they are losing control as they begin to enter a state of relaxation. Meditation is somewhat more likely than other relaxation techniques to produce this response.

Prerecorded Relaxation Tapes

Many cassette tapes present excellent relaxation instructions. Some bookstores stock relaxation tapes, or you can contact these sources for catalogs:

- *Stress Management Research Associates, P.O. Box 2232-B, Houston, TX 77251; 713-890-8575*

- *BMA Audio Cassettes, 200 Park Avenue South, New York, NY 10003, 800-221-3966*

- *New Harbinger Publications, 5674 Shattuck Avenue, Oakland, CA 94609; 800-748-6273*

Choosing and Using a Relaxation Technique

As we saw above, you can choose the relaxation method or combination of methods that feels most comfortable and works for you. In addition, you get to choose when to use the technique. It is best to set aside time for one or two relaxation sessions a day, to increase your skill and lower your level of physical tension. The longer you practice, the more proficient you will become and the better you will be able to use the relaxation response to cope with stress and anxiety. You will find that your relaxation sessions take less time as you learn the skills.

Consider learning the tense-and-release method as an initial investment. It requires more time and effort than some of the other techniques. But the contrast you observe between tension and relaxation will help you learn and use passive relaxation methods.

In addition to planned relaxation times, treat yourself to brief periods of relaxation throughout the day. Although you can relax more deeply with your eyes closed, you can achieve effective relaxation with your eyes open. In that way, you can secretly use relaxation methods during a meeting or other social function. With practice, you can induce a pleasant sense of relaxation to spread through your body in just six seconds — the time between phone rings. In fact, quick relaxation periods are sometimes called *six-second tranquilizers.*

The average American adult spends forty minutes a day waiting. We wait at stop signs, for cashiers, meetings, and TV commercials, and on hold during phone calls. Instead of feeling frustrated by waiting, use the time as an opportunity for a six-second tranquilizer. Here are some ideas for incorporating relaxation into your everyday routine:

- *When the telephone rings, don't answer it right away. Instead, wait the six seconds before the next ring while you find tension and breathe it away.*

- *Relax while you are waiting at an elevator or a red light. If you have more than six seconds to wait, enjoy the relaxation for as long as you have.*

- *Put a tiny piece of colored tape on your watch. Whenever you check the time, use the tape as a cue reminding you to relax.*

- *Put pieces of tape on your IN basket at work and your refrigerator at home. Use the tape as signals to relax.*

- *Each time you sit down, breathe away your tension.*

Relaxation at bedtime can help reduce insomnia, as we will see in Chapter 15.

COGNITIVE TECHNIQUES

In the previous chapter, we saw how our thoughts can contribute to depression. Similarly, distorted thinking and irrational beliefs can exacerbate stress and anxiety.

We have seen that cognitive therapy can be used — either with a professional or in self-help methods — to alleviate depression. Cognitive therapy can also help reduce our feelings of stress and anxiety. In the remainder of this chapter we will see how.

The things we tell ourselves — or *self-talk* — can make us feel either anxious or calm. Let's look at some typical anxiety-raising thoughts we might experience. After each anxious thought, look at the alternative calming thoughts we can use in the same situation.

THOUGHTS THAT INCREASE STRESS AND ANXIETY	*CORRESPONDING THOUGHTS THAT REDUCE STRESS AND ANXIETY*
"I've got so much to do!"	"I'll start the most important project first."
"Don't blow it."	"I'll just do my best."
"This is too much for me."	"I know I can handle it."
"I'm getting all tense again."	"I feel some tension. I'll just relax the muscles that are tight."
"I shouldn't be afraid."	"A little anxiety is normal. And it motivates me to do my best."
"I can't stand it!"	"This is only temporary. I can stand it. I've been through worse."

"It's not fair."	"Bad things happen to everybody."
"That jerk!"	"Getting mad won't help. Just stay cool and deal with the problem."
"I'll get even."	"Take some deep breaths and chill out. This battle isn't worth it."
"He thinks I'm a pushover."	"What he thinks doesn't matter."
"I'll never get to work through this traffic."	"Traffic is just part of the deal if I choose to live in the city."
"I won't let that bastard cut me off."	"He's an unsafe driver. I'll be cool and stay away from him."

Notice that the last five thoughts above relate specifically to anger, one type of stress response. The others involve more generalized stress or anxiety responses.

You *choose* self-talk that makes you anxious or angry. You can just as easily choose self-talk that calms you. Try to become aware of thoughts that make you angry or anxious. When you identify an anxiety-raising thought, *change it*. Remember, negative self-talk is just a habit. You aren't born saying these things to yourself; you *learn* to think them. What you have learned you can unlearn, because you're in charge of your thoughts.

You can make an effort to notice when your thoughts are anxiety-provoking and to counter negative self-talk with positive alternatives. If you regularly make this effort, your thoughts and beliefs will become less anxious. You will change the way you think *and feel*.

PUTTING IT ALL TOGETHER

Learning these techniques and substituting them for the habits of a lifetime is not an overnight process. Change takes time and practice. But if you invest a little time, you will reduce your day-to-day levels of stress and anxiety. On those occasions when your stress and anxiety reach high levels, you will have the tools for managing them. And if you reduce your level of tension during the day and evening, you will become less tense at bedtime.

RECOMMENDED SELF-HELP BOOKS

Many books present further information on managing stress and anxiety. The following three are among the most useful currently available.

- Edward Charlesworth and Ronald Nathan, *Stress Management: A Comprehensive Guide to Wellness* (New York: Random House, 1985).
  This book thoroughly explores relaxation methods, assertiveness, time management, exercise, nutrition, and other methods of stress management.

- Martha Davis, Elizabeth Eshelman, and Matthew McKay, *The Relaxation and Stress Reduction Workbook* (Oakland, Calif.: New Harbinger, 1988).
  This is a practical guide to methods of reducing stress's negative impact.

- David Burns, *The Feeling Good Handbook* (New York: Plume, 1990).
  In this acclaimed sequel to *Feeling Good* (see page 157), the methods of cognitive therapy are applied to anxiety disorders and other problems.

PROFESSIONAL HELP

If you experience high levels of stress or anxiety, you may want to seek help from a mental-health professional or stress-management consultant. Specific training and experience in cognitive and behavioral methods are more important than the type of degree the professional holds.

The last section of Chapter 9 reviews different ways to find and choose a qualified mental-health professional. Use one of those methods. Make sure that you are clear about the specialist's approach, that it makes sense to you, and that you feel comfortable with it.

11

Sleep-Wake Rhythms and Sunday-Night Insomnia

MOST OF US SLEEP AT NIGHT AND STAY AWAKE DURING THE day. It's obvious enough that our sleep-wake schedule pretty much follows the rhythm of the sun shining on the rotating earth: We stay active when the sun is in the sky and sleep when it's dark. Because our sleep-wake rhythm goes along with the twenty-four-hour solar day, you might guess that this rhythm is linked with the cycle of darkness and light. And it is — but not precisely.

In humans and other mammals, hundreds of physical functions follow daily rhythms. These natural biological patterns are called *circadian rhythms*, from the Latin *circa*, meaning "about," and *dies*, meaning "a day."

In 1866 it was discovered that body temperature rises in the morning and drops at night. Modern research on circadian rhythms began only in the 1950s, and it has increased dramatically since about 1980. Scientists have discovered that such body processes as hormone production, cell multiplication, and mental performance ebb and flow with the cycle of light and darkness. Light enters the retinas of the eyes and travels along a neural pathway to the hypothalamus, where it influences the timing of the body clock. This biological clock prepares us for sleep at night and for wakefulness in the day.

Our circadian rhythm is regulated by a group of nerve cells in the brain's hypothalamus, a structure the size of a fingertip that also is involved in many complex behaviors: eating, temperature regulation, emotional responses, sexual behavior, and aggressive behavior. This interesting area in the brain is the site of our biological clock.

The science of *chronobiology* studies the rhythms of life that are regulated by biological clocks. In numerous studies, chronobiologists have established that our internal biological rhythms strongly affect alertness and mental performance. For most of us, the low point of these abilities is between 1:00 and 5:00 A.M., when our body temperature is low and we are least alert. The Three-Mile Island and *Exxon Valdez* accidents and the Chernobyl and Bhopal disasters all occurred during this period. Human error was implicated in all four incidents.

OUR TWENTY-FIVE-HOUR INTERNAL DAY

In many different time-isolation experiments, more than five hundred human subjects have spent up to six months in caves, cellars, and soundproof windowless apartments. These settings are totally isolated from the day-night cycle. Subjects have no access to clocks and to such social cues to the actual time outside as televisions, radios, and telephones. They are permitted to turn lights on and off and to sleep and wake when they please. (In most time-isolation experiments, naps are prohibited because a nap can throw off the body's circadian rhythm.)

When left on their own to stay awake and to sleep according to their own internal cues, most adult subjects show a curious phenomenon. They shift to a *twenty-five-*

Circadian Rhythms Are **Not** Biorhythms

The pervasive circadian rhythms found in most of our body functions should not be confused with the pseudoscience of "biorhythms."

Biorhythms are purported to forecast the quality of changing abilities in an individual based on the date and hour of the person's birth. According to biorhythm enthusiasts, much of our behavior is governed by a thirty-three-day intellectual cycle, a twenty-eight-day emotional cycle, and a twenty-three-day physical cycle. The interaction of these cycles is alleged to influence the quality of our performance.

The idea of biorhythms began about a hundred years ago. The concept was revived during the 1930s and again in the 1970s, when biorhythm charting services were heavily advertised. Simple computers that generated biorhythm charts appeared in shopping malls and other locations. By depositing a quarter, customers could learn the days their levels of mental, emotional, and physical functioning were predicted to arrive at peaks and troughs. In the nationally televised pregame show for the 1978 Super Bowl, sports announcers revealed that the biorhythm charts of the two teams predicted that the Denver Broncos would defeat the Dallas Cowboys.

Biorhythm lore is intuitively appealing because of its apparent simplicity and logic. However, in a series of rigorous studies examining biorhythmic predictions of accidents, deaths, and athletic performance, biorhythms were found to be completely unrelated to such events. (The Cowboys, unaware of—and therefore unaffected by—their supposedly problematic biorhythms, went on to trounce the Broncos, 27–10.)

People have good days and bad days, but biorhythms do not predict when they occur. Biorhythms correlate with behavior only when a person has seen a biorhythm chart predicting a certain type of day and thereby is primed to expect that kind of day. This pattern results from the fact that our thoughts and expectations can influence our feelings and our behavior, as we saw in Chapters 9 and 10.

hour day. Each day they fall asleep and awaken about an hour later than the day before. So if a subject's initial sleep schedule is 11:00 P.M. to 7:00 A.M., his or her sleep time will shift on the second night to midnight to 8:00 A.M. and on the third night to 1:00 A.M. to 9:00 A.M. This tendency to desynchronize from the twenty-four-hour solar day and follow the internal clock's drift to later hours is known as *free-running.*

Although our natural biological cycle is twenty-five hours long, our internal clock adjusts readily to the twenty-four-hour day. In most parts of the country, we reset our circadian clocks by one hour every spring and fall. This occurs in the spring, when we set our clocks forward one hour to change to daylight saving time, and in the fall, when we set them back an hour to return to standard time.

Because the internal clock tends to run toward a longer day, it is more difficult to adjust to spring's time change, which requires us to go to bed and get up an hour earlier than before. In fact, during the week after the spring change to daylight saving time, an 11 percent increase in traffic accidents has been documented. In contrast, we adjust easily to the autumn change to standard time, because in relation to solar time we are going to bed and getting up later than before. Appendix 4 shows that the same phenomenon occurs during travel: We adjust more easily to westbound than eastbound travel, because with westbound travel we go to bed and get up later than before.

Similarly, we all need to "set back" our internal twenty-five-hour clocks *every day* by one hour, to keep ourselves in time with our natural and social environments. We synchronize ourselves to the twenty-four-hour day by such routines as regular wake-up times, exposure to sunlight on the way to work, regular mealtimes, and routinely going to bed after the late news. These external cues that help us keep in synchronism with the twenty-four-hour day are called *zeitgebers,* from the German *zeit,* meaning "time," and *geber,* which means "giver."

As long as we use zeitgebers every day, we will keep our internal clocks synchronized to the twenty-four-hour day. But if we don't keep regular routines, we can cause ourselves problems.

WHEN CIRCADIAN CLOCKS BECOME CONFUSED

Many people with chronic insomnia vary their bedtimes and waking times. On a night when they experience insomnia, the following morning they sleep in late to make up for the sleep they lost. That day they may try to nap, again to make up for lost sleep. That evening they may go to bed at an early hour, before they're drowsy. Then they can't fall asleep, or they fall asleep but awaken when their sleep becomes shallower within a few hours.

Sporadic changing of bedtimes and rising times throws off the body's natural circadian rhythm. If you have a stable sleep-wake rhythm, your body will become sleepy at about the same time each night. In contrast, if you try to make up lost sleep by going to bed early, napping, and sleeping in late, you will destabilize your body's circadian rhythm. This can worsen and perpetuate an insomnia problem.

Extreme cases of this kind of problem are diagnosed as the circadian disorder of *irregular sleep-wake pattern*. This pattern is most often shown by jobless or retired people and by people who work at home on their own schedule. People in these situations do not have their sleep-wake rhythms anchored to the zeitgeber of regular job hours. Some people with this problem live their lives in a haze of drowsiness, naps, and fragmented sleep.

There is a simple way to stabilize an erratic circadian system: *Establish a regular sleep-wake schedule, and follow it seven days a week.* Go to bed and get up at the same time each day. If you feel that you must sleep in on weekends, sleep at most one hour later than usual, and open the curtains to expose yourself to daylight as soon as you awaken.

You can take several other steps to stabilize your sleep-wake rhythm: Avoid naps. Be active during the day, and make an effort to do aerobic exercise several times a week. Expose yourself to sunlight.

MORNING PEOPLE AND NIGHT PEOPLE

The terms "lark" and "owl" are used by chronobiologists to describe individuals who reach a peak of alertness and performance at different times of the day. Owls — or night people — function best in the evening. Their internal clocks run on a cycle longer than the adult average of twenty-five hours, and they reach a body-temperature peak later than the average of around 6:00 P.M.

In contrast, larks — or morning people — are at their peak times early in the day. Their internal clocks tend to run on a cycle shorter than the adult average of twenty-five hours, and they reach a body-temperature peak earlier than average. With increasing age, people tend more to become larks, as we will see later in the chapter.

Most of us are not strongly predisposed in either direction, and have no more than slight to moderate tendencies toward early or late hours.

Below is a questionnaire you can use to determine the direction of your body rhythms, as well as how strongly they tend that way.

LARK-OWL SCALE*

1. What time would you choose to get up if you were free to plan your day?
   A. 5:00 A.M. to 6:00 A.M.
   B. 6:00 A.M. to 7:30 A.M.
   C. 7:30 A.M. to 10:00 A.M.
   D. 10:00 A.M. to 11:00 A.M.
   E. 11:00 A.M. to noon

2. You have to attend to some important business, for which you want to feel at the peak of your mental powers. When would you prefer this meeting to take place?
   A. 8:00 A.M. to 10:00 A.M.
   B. 11:00 A.M. to 1:00 P.M.
   C. 3:00 P.M. to 5:00 P.M.
   D. 7:00 P.M. to 9:00 P.M.

3. What time would you choose to go to bed if you were entirely free to plan your evening?
   A. 8:00 P.M. to 9:00 P.M.
   B. 9:00 P.M. to 10:15 P.M.
   C. 10:15 P.M. to 12:30 A.M.
   D. 12:30 A.M. to 1:45 A.M.
   E. 1:45 A.M. to 3:00 A.M.

4. A friend suggests jogging with you, beginning at 7:00 A.M. How would you feel at this time?
   A. In good form
   B. In reasonable form
   C. You would find it difficult
   D. You would find it very difficult

5. You have some physical work to do. At what time would you feel able to do it best?
   A. 8:00 A.M. to 10:00 A.M.
   B. 11:00 A.M. to 1:00 P.M.
   C. 3:00 P.M. to 5:00 P.M.
   D. 7:00 P.M. to 9:00 P.M.

6. You have to go to bed at 11:00 P.M. How would you feel?
   A. Not at all tired, unable to get to sleep quickly
   B. A little tired, unlikely to get to sleep quickly
   C. Fairly tired, likely to get to sleep quickly
   D. Very tired, very likely to get to sleep quickly

7. When you have been up for half an hour on a normal working day, how do you feel?
   A. Very tired
   B. Fairly tired
   C. Fairly refreshed
   D. Very refreshed

8. At what time of the day do you feel best?
   A. 8:00 A.M. to 10:00 A.M.
   B. 11:00 A.M. to 1:00 P.M.
   C. 3:00 P.M. to 5:00 P.M.
   D. 7:00 P.M. to 9:00 P.M.

9. Another friend suggests jogging with you, beginning at 10:00 P.M. How would you now feel?
   A. In good form
   B. In reasonable form
   C. You would find it difficult
   D. You would find it very difficult

Now score your answers. Add up the points for the 9 questions.

1.	2.	3.
A = 1	A = 1	A = 1
B = 2	B = 2	B = 2
C = 3	C = 3	C = 3
D = 4	D = 4	D = 4
E = 5		E = 5

4.	5.	6.
A = 1	A = 1	A = 4
B = 2	B = 2	B = 3
C = 3	C = 3	C = 2
D = 4	D = 4	D = 1

7.	8.	9.
A = 4	A = 1	A = 4
B = 3	B = 2	B = 3
C = 2	C = 3	C = 2
D = 1	D = 4	D = 1

---

*Adapted from *Your Body Clock*, James Waterhouse, David Minors, and Maureen Waterhouse (Oxford, England: Oxford University Press, 1990). Reprinted by permission of Oxford University Press. This book by two British chronobiologists and a science writer is an excellent source of information about biological rhythms, night work, and jet lag.

INTERPRETING YOUR SCORE

Your score can range from 9 to 38. This is only a guide, of course, but your score can be interpreted as follows:

9–15 Definitely a lark
16–20 Moderately a lark

21–26 Neither a lark nor an owl; intermediate type
27–31 Moderately an owl
32–38 Definitely an owl

CHANGES IN OUR BODY CLOCKS WITH AGE

Our circadian rhythms show predictable changes as we grow older.

During old age the internal rhythms of about a third of people over sixty-five become shorter than the twenty-four-hour day, causing them to become larks, or morning people. This pattern is more likely to emerge among women than men. These people tend to become sleepy and go to bed early in the evening. If they go to bed by 8:00 or 9:00 P.M., they awaken by 3:00 or 4:00 A.M., and are unable to sleep any longer. For these older adults, a regular bedtime is the most important zeitgeber to keep the body clock synchronized to a twenty-four-hour day. Other suggestions are given on page 204 under "Shifting a Morning Person's Circadian Rhythms."

Another change occurs in old age: The daily ups and downs of the sleep-wake rhythm become flatter and less pronounced. Compared with when we were younger, our sleep is more shallow, and we lie awake in bed more at night. During the day we are less active and we tend to nap. The polarity between nighttime sleep and daytime wakefulness decreases as night and day blend together.

The core body temperature of a young adult is about two degrees Fahrenheit lower during the night than during the day. This variation reflects a strong daily sleep-wake rhythm. In contrast, a seventy-five-year-old shows a temperature difference of just a half degree or less.

Some older adults adapt comfortably to the changes caused by a flatter circadian rhythm. Those who want to strengthen their circadian rhythms and sleep better at night should avoid naps, expose themselves to sunlight, exercise during the day, and stay awake until a regular bedtime.

THREE WAYS TO SHIFT A NIGHT PERSON'S
CIRCADIAN RHYTHMS

Sometimes night people's sleep-wake pattern can disrupt their social and occupational functioning. An extreme form of a night person's sleep-wake pattern is called *delayed sleep phase syndrome.*

People with delayed sleep phase syndrome are most a-lert late in the evening, and they go to bed very late at night. If they shift their bedtimes to an earlier hour, they cannot fall asleep until their usual late bedtimes. Conse-quently, these people have a hard time waking up and getting up for school or daytime jobs. Their sleep-wake rhythm is so delayed that a conventional 6:00 or 7:00 A.M. waking time feels like the middle of the night according to their internal clocks.

People with delayed sleep phase syndrome sleep well if they can follow their strong circadian preference for very late hours. In fact, on weekends and during vacations they usually drift to a later sleep schedule, falling asleep long after midnight and getting up around noon. However, they sleep little if they try to follow the conventional hours of a day worker. Delayed sleep phase syndrome causes about 10 percent of chronic insomnia cases. People with this problem have difficulty falling asleep rather than staying asleep.

If you are an extreme night owl and you want to adjust your body rhythm to an earlier schedule, there are three approaches to consider. The most effective method is *light therapy.*

LIGHT THERAPY

This procedure, also known as *phototherapy,* is a relatively new intervention that now is used widely to treat disorders of circadian rhythms. Research on light therapy is in the mainstream of science and is being conducted at many universities. Much of the leading work in light therapy is being done by the research group at Harvard Medical School's Center for Circadian and Sleep Disorders Medicine.

In light therapy, you expose yourself to bright light early in the morning. The light source must be at least 2,500 lux. This is five to ten times brighter than ordinary room light, which is not intense enough to affect your circadian clock. You need to be exposed to 2,500 lux for one to two hours.

One way to expose yourself to light is simply to go outside. Shortly after sunrise, daylight ranges from 2,500 lux to 8,000 lux, depending on whether the morning is cloudy or clear. A walk or drive of twenty to sixty minutes — such as a commute to work — can be effective, although some people need exposure for up to two hours. If you don't wear sunglasses, you will receive a stronger light stimulus.

A faster way to expose yourself to light is to use a compact light box. These range in intensity from 2,500 to 10,000 lux. If the light source is 10,000 lux, exposure usually needs to last for only fifteen to thirty minutes.

The Society for Light Treatment and Biological Rhythms is a nonprofit association that publishes a newsletter and other information. You can contact this group at P.O. Box 478, Wilsonville, OR 97070; 503-694-2404. It can provide the names of practitioners in your area experienced in light therapy. It can also provide a complete list of companies that sell light boxes and other products, such as visors with high-intensity lights tucked beneath the brim.

These are a few of the companies that will send you brochures and literature about light therapy:

- *Ambulatory Monitoring, 731 Saw Mill River Road, Ardsley, NY 10502; 800-341-0066*

- *Apollo Light Systems, 352 West 1060th South, Orem, UT 84058; 800-545-9667*

- *The Sun Box Company, 19217 Orbit Drive, Gaithersburg, MD 20879; 800-548-3968*

In 1993 the price of a light box averages four hundred and fifty dollars. Some insurance companies reimburse the cost of a light box if a physician certifies it as medically necessary. (Light therapy is used also to treat seasonal affective disorder, a type of depression that occurs during the winter because of reduced sunlight. In some cases it may help other depressive disorders as well.)

You can read, write, exercise, watch TV, or do anything you want during light therapy. To avoid eye damage, don't look directly into an artificial light source, just as you wouldn't look at the sun. But don't wear sunglasses to ease the glare, because the light has to enter the retina of your eyes and travel to the brain's internal clock to be effective. Some drugs cause light sensitivity, so ask your doctor or pharmacist whether this may be a factor with any medications you are taking. If you have any disorder of the eyes or skin, consult your physician before beginning light therapy.

You can augment the effectiveness of morning light therapy by avoiding bright lights late in the day. Wear dark, wraparound sunglasses when you are outside in the hours before sunset. This will prevent daylight from entering your eyes and cuing your brain that it is time to be awake and alert.

If light therapy works for you, improvement will appear within two to four days. However, you may need to continue the treatment for a month, to stabilize your new, earlier sleep-wake rhythm. Then see if you can continue your early schedule without light therapy. Some people relapse when they stop light treatment, and they need to keep it up indefinitely.

CHRONOTHERAPY

A second way to change the late schedule of extreme night people with delayed sleep phase syndrome is *chronotherapy*. This process works quite well, but it has been done rarely since about 1990, because light therapy is a simpler way to reset circadian rhythms.

Chronotherapy is the process of pushing forward your bedtime and waking time, until your sleep-wake schedule matches the schedule you need to follow. In contrast with moving backward to an earlier schedule, chronotherapy works with the normal internal preference for a later, longer day.

In chronotherapy a person who normally sleeps from 5:00 A.M. to 1:00 P.M. delays the sleep period three hours, to 8:00 A.M. to 4:00 P.M. on the first day, then 11:00 A.M. to 7:00 P.M. on the second day, then 2:00 P.M. to 10:00 P.M., and so on. This makes for a series of twenty-seven-hour days. The three-hour daily shift continues for about six days, until the person goes "around the clock" to a more conventional sleep schedule.

Of course, the process needs to be done during vacation or some other time when the person doesn't face the demands of a regular schedule. It is necessary to shield the bedroom from sunlight when the person sleeps during the day.

Chronotherapy can be done even faster, by advancing the sleep schedule four or five hours each day. In this way, the circadian clock can be reset over four days.

SLEEP DEPRIVATION

A third method to move to an earlier sleep-wake schedule is to use all-night sleep deprivation to make yourself sleepy at an earlier hour. Begin by staying up all night on a Friday or Saturday. Don't nap the following day, so your body will be sleepy earlier than usual that night. Then adjust your sleep schedule by going to bed and getting up earlier. This procedure has been effective in helping night owls shift their bedtimes and wake-up times ninety minutes earlier. Depending on how much earlier you want to shift your sleep schedule, you may need to repeat the procedure over a second or even a third weekend.

SHIFTING A MORNING PERSON'S CIRCADIAN RHYTHMS

We have seen that the body's circadian clock sometimes speeds up in old age, shifting from a twenty-five-hour rhythm to one shorter than twenty-four hours. A short circadian rhythm causes the person to fall asleep early in the evening and consequently to awaken much too early in the morning. This condition, the opposite of a night owl's delayed sleep phase syndrome, is called *advanced sleep phase syndrome.*

Someone with this problem should resist going to bed until late in the evening. One way to maintain wakefulness during the evening is to use light therapy. People with advanced sleep phase syndrome should expose themselves to bright light during the late afternoon and early evening. In the spring and summer, simply going outside in the sunlight is best. At other times of the year, exposure to a light box around 8:00 P.M. can be effective. At 2,500 lux, one to two hours of exposure are needed. At 10,000 lux, just fifteen to thirty minutes are enough. It also is helpful to avoid morning sunlight and to wear dark, wraparound sunglasses outdoors before noon.

This procedure can help older adults — who often fall asleep and awaken too early — to shift their circadian rhythms to a more conventional schedule. This treatment is precisely the opposite of the one that younger people with delayed sleep phase syndrome use to shift their sleep schedule in the reverse direction. (Early-morning awakening associated with depression is sometimes improved by this form of light therapy.)

Advanced sleep phase syndrome also has been treated by chronotherapy, in which people go to bed earlier each day, until they go "around the clock" and finally fall asleep and wake up later than when they started the treatment. However, light therapy is much simpler and more likely to be effective.

SUNDAY-NIGHT INSOMNIA

Some people experience insomnia only on Sunday nights. Others have trouble sleeping throughout the week, but Sunday night is the worst. Still others say that at first they had only Sunday-night insomnia but then began to have trouble sleeping on other nights as well. Let's look at the cause and the solution of this common problem.

On weekends, many of us stay up past our usual bedtimes and turn off our alarm clocks. If we alter our sleep routines in this way, we encourage our sleep-wake cycles to follow the body's natural drift to a twenty-five-hour day. As we have seen, this pattern is called free-running. It feels good on Friday and Saturday nights, as well as Saturday and Sunday mornings. But it causes a problem on Sunday night.

Let's say you normally go to bed at 11:00 P.M. and get up at 7:00 A.M. On Friday night you follow your body's preference and stay up an hour later, until midnight. On Saturday morning you sleep in until eight. By then your internal clock is an hour behind your bedside clock because you went to bed and got up an hour later than usual.

On Saturday night you again follow your body's preference and stay up until 1:00 A.M. — an hour later than Friday night and two hours later than your usual 11:00 P.M. bedtime. On Sunday morning you sleep in until 9:00 — an hour later than on Saturday morning, and two hours later than your usual wake-up time of 7:00 A.M.

After a weekend of going to bed later and sleeping late in the mornings, your internal clock is two hours behind your bedside clock by Sunday night. And if you nap on Sunday afternoon, your internal clock falls *another* hour or so behind. Now, if you try to go to bed at your usual 11:00 P.M. bedtime, your body will feel as if it were two or three hours earlier, or only 8:00 or 9:00 P.M. That's why you can't fall asleep.

Your internal biological clock will finally catch up with your bedside clock at 1:00 or 2:00 A.M. But by then you've been lying in bed for two or three hours worrying about the fact that you can't sleep. And because it's Sunday night, you're probably thinking about the approaching workweek as well. It's natural to be a little sad that the weekend's over; but from that rational feeling it's easy to jump to the false assumption that you can't sleep *because* you're thinking about work.

So now you're worried about three things: (1) the fact that you can't sleep; (2) the impending workweek; (3) your perception that you must be *so* worried about the workweek that the worry is causing your insomnia. With all this running around in your head, you may have a hard time getting drowsy even when your internal clock finally schedules you for sleep at 1:00 or 2:00 A.M.

And when the alarm goes off at 7:00, your body will still be two or three hours behind, feeling as though it's only 4:00 or 5:00 A.M. No wonder it's hard to get up on Monday mornings.

Going to bed late and sleeping in late on weekends — and then returning to your normal hours after the weekend — can produce a state of time confusion in the body that is identical to jet lag. If you're a New Yorker who wakes up at 7:00 A.M. during the workweek and at 9:00 A.M. on weekends, it is as if each week you flew west across two time zones to spend the weekend in Denver. During the weekend you sleep on Mountain Time rather than Eastern Time. Making this first change is easy, because it incorporates into your schedule the

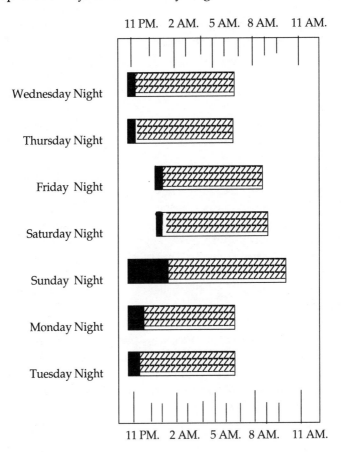

11 PM.   2 AM.   5 AM.   8 AM.   11 AM.

Wednesday Night

Thursday Night

Friday Night

Saturday Night

Sunday Night

Monday Night

Tuesday Night

11 PM.   2 AM.   5 AM.   8 AM.   11 AM.

Awake in bed
ZZZZZ Asleep in bed

FIGURE 11–1
THE SLEEPING PATTERN OF SUNDAY-NIGHT
INSOMNIA

Notice how long it takes the person to fall asleep on Sunday night after having slept in all weekend. (Adapted with permission from Thomas Coates and Carl Thoresen, *How to Sleep Better* [Englewood Cliffs, N.J.: Prentice-Hall, 1977].)

body's natural tendency to drift to later hours. But the *second* change, returning to the workweek's 7:00 A.M. wake-up time, is the same as though you had suddenly flown back from the mountain time zone to the eastern time zone. Varying your sleep hours over the weekend induces a kind of jet lag without flying anywhere.

THE SUNDAY BLUES

Many people are so troubled by Sunday-night insomnia that during the afternoon they begin to feel its harbinger. As the weekend winds down from the euphoria of Friday night, through Saturday and then Sunday, only Sunday evening remains before the return to school or work. Around this time, many of us experience a downward mood swing toward malaise or melancholy. The flip side of TGIF — thank God it's Friday — makes its appearance around midafternoon as the Sunday blues.

The Sunday blues are complex and not well understood. But they seem to be the worst in people who have trouble sleeping on Sunday night. The Sunday blues often accompany the realization that within hours will come the weekly bout with Sunday-night insomnia. Even people who enjoy their jobs and the company of their co-workers can get the Sunday blues.

THE SOLUTION

Curing Sunday-night insomnia will give you two positive side effects: You will reduce the impact of its precursor, the Sunday blues, as well as its camp follower, the Monday blahs. And the best cure for Sunday-night insomnia is prevention. *Simply get up at your regular weekday wakeup time on Saturday and Sunday mornings.*

On Friday and Saturday nights it's best to go to bed near your regular bedtime, but this isn't essential. What is essential is to keep to your regular wake-up time on Saturday and Sunday mornings. If you go to sleep late and consequently sleep less on Friday and Saturday nights, you may feel a little drowsy at first when you get up at your regular time on Saturday and Sunday mornings — but your biological clock won't be thrown off. You'll have more time to read the paper, take a walk, or otherwise enjoy the morning. It is a uniquely invigorating feeling to be awake on a Sunday morning at your weekday rising time, knowing that you have a whole day ahead of you — not a day shortened by sleeping in — and that your day won't end with Sunday-night insomnia.

If you feel that you *must* sleep in on weekends, there is an alternate (though less effective) way to minimize Sunday-night insomnia. Allow yourself to sleep in on weekend mornings, but no more than one hour later than your weekday rising time, and expose yourself to sunlight as soon as you awaken: Take a walk outdoors or sit near a bright window. Then, on Sunday night, don't aim for your regular weekday bedtime. Instead stay up one hour later. Because you slept one hour later on Sunday morning, your body won't be ready to sleep until one hour later than usual. If you follow this schedule, you will sleep about one hour less than usual on Sunday night. But as Chapter 1 showed, losing sleep won't hurt your health or your daytime performance.

Whichever solution you use, if you are susceptible to Sunday-night insomnia, it is best not to nap on the weekend — especially on Sunday — because a daytime nap can throw off your circadian rhythm, further delaying the hour you become sleepy and cutting into your nighttime sleep appetite. (There is more on the subject of naps in Chapter 14.)

If you still find yourself experiencing Sunday-night insomnia, don't stay in bed and try to force sleep. When your circadian rhythms tell your body that it's still time to be awake, you can't override those internal signals. Instead, get out of bed and read, watch TV, or do something else until you become drowsy.

Part IV offers many specific recommendations for inducing sleep and improving sleep quality. Use these techniques especially on Sunday if you tend to have Sunday-night insomnia. (For example, on Sunday it is a very good idea to get in the habit of exercising during the late afternoon or early evening.)

NEW RESEARCH

Exciting research is being conducted on *melatonin*, a hormone secreted by the brain during darkness. Melatonin serves as a cue to the body that it is time to sleep. Its secretion is suppressed by light therapy.

Melatonin has been synthesized in the laboratory, and much work has been done on its effects on body clocks. In a 1992 article in the journal *Chronobiology International*, psychiatrist Alfred Lewy and his research group at Oregon Health Sciences University demonstrated that synthetic melatonin can shift circadian rhythms in humans. By 1997 melatonin will likely be available by prescription. Synthetic melatonin may help counteract problems associated with advanced and delayed sleep phase syndromes, seasonal affective disorder, shift work (Appendix 3), and jet lag (Appendix 4).

12

Conditioned Insomnia: When Your Bed Keeps You Awake

SOUND SLEEPERS HAVE LEARNED TO ASSOCIATE DROWSINESS with their bedrooms and their beds. For them, lying down in bed serves as a signal that begins to induce sleep. This association of sleep with bed develops over years of falling asleep at bedtime. Good sleepers typically sleep better in their own beds than anywhere else, because they associate their beds with drowsiness.

Insomnia sufferers, in contrast, become tense when they lie in bed. They have lain awake so many sleepless nights that they have learned to associate frustrated wakefulness with their bed and bedroom. Simply put, their bed and bedroom remind them of their past bouts with insomnia.

For good sleepers, the bed serves as a stimulus for the sleep response. But for poor sleepers, the bed is a stimulus for alertness. They have learned — or been *conditioned* — to associate arousal and insomnia with their beds, so their sleep problem is called *conditioned insomnia*, or *learned insomnia*.

Conditioned insomnia usually begins when sleep is disrupted by stress, illness, or any other factor. After the initial cause of sleeplessness has gone away, the person continues to have insomnia because of the learned associations between wakefulness and the bedroom. Some people are more susceptible to conditioned insomnia than others. Those who develop conditioned insomnia tend to be more tense or "high-strung" than other people.

People with conditioned insomnia often say that they can hardly stay awake on an easy chair or couch in the living room, but as soon as they go into their bedrooms, they feel wide-awake. You may have conditioned insomnia if you sleep better in your living room or in a hotel room than in your own bedroom.

If your sleep has been disrupted by one of the factors discussed in Chapters 5 through 11, the insomnia may persist even after you have solved the sleep problem that caused it originally. Conditioned insomnia can make your sleeplessness continue because you have learned to associate your bed and bedroom with wakefulness. Fortunately, there is an effective method to undo the maladaptive learning of conditioned insomnia and learn to associate your bed and bedroom with sleep.

HOW TO UNLEARN CONDITIONED INSOMNIA

At Northwestern University in the 1970s psychologist Richard Bootzin developed a highly successful set of procedures for overcoming conditioned insomnia. They help you unlearn the conditioned response of arousal and wakefulness you experience when lying in bed.

Research has established clearly that we are influenced by associations in which we pair certain kinds of behavior with certain situations. For example, you reach for a cigarette when you drink beer or coffee, feel excited when you are in a stadium full of sports fans, or experience anxiety when the phone rings in the middle of the night. The situation (or stimulus) becomes a cue or signal for the behavior (or response) to occur. This learning principle is called *stimulus control.*

Stimulus control can help you unlearn the association of bed with anxiety. The procedures pair the bed and bedroom with rapid sleep onset. In this way you become reconditioned, so that you come to associate your bed with drowsiness and sleep. The act of lying in bed then serves as a cue to induce sleep.

There are five steps in the stimulus-control method:

1. Go to bed only when you feel sleepy, no matter how late the hour. This step will help ensure that you feel sleepy when you climb into bed. Feeling drowsy at bedtime makes it likely that you will fall asleep fast. And falling asleep fast will help you learn to associate your bed with drowsiness and sleep. This in turn will cause you to fall asleep more quickly in the future.

2. Use your bed only for sleeping. Don't read, watch television, worry, or do anything else in bed. This step will help you break a learned association of your bed with sleeplessness, and substitute an association of bed with sleep.

   There is one exception. It's all right to make love in bed.

   If you tend to worry, ruminate about the day's events, or plan for tomorrow while you're in bed, spend some quiet time doing these activities in another room *before* you go to bed. There is more about this idea in Chapter 14.

3. If you don't fall asleep in ten to twenty minutes, get up and go to another room. Don't watch the clock as the minutes pass because clock watching makes it harder to relax and fall asleep. The point is to get out of bed if sleep doesn't come easily, to break the association between the bed and frustrated arousal.

If you don't soon fall asleep and you then get up, don't return to bed until you feel really sleepy again. If you still can't fall asleep readily, get up again. Repeat this procedure as often as necessary through the night.

When you awaken during the night, give yourself ten or twenty minutes to fall back asleep. If you don't return to sleep easily, get out of bed.

To make this step easier to follow, keep a robe and slippers handy, have a book ready to read or something else to do in another room, and during the winter months arrange beforehand to keep another room reasonably warm during the night.

4. Use your alarm clock to get up at the same time every morning, regardless of how little sleep you got the night before. If you anchor your sleep-wake rhythm to a regular rising time, that rhythm will stabilize. A stable sleep-wake rhythm will cause you to become sleepy at the same time each night.

5. Don't nap during the day. Napping to make up for lost sleep will destabilize your sleep-wake rhythms and make you less sleepy at bedtime that night. If you feel drowsy during the day, take a shower rather than nap. Or take a brisk walk; as noted in Chapter 9, aerobic exercise actually counteracts fatigue and restores energy.

During the first night of the stimulus control procedure, you may need to get out of bed five times or more. You may not sleep at all, and you will feel tired the next day. At this point you might think that the remedy is worse than the original problem.

It takes determination to keep up with the procedure. But by the second, third, or fourth night, sleep deprivation will cause your body to fall asleep more quickly. Most people need about two weeks to undo completely the maladaptive learning of conditioned insomnia. If you stick with the plan, you will begin again to associate your bed and bedroom with sleep.

Stimulus control is easy to understand, but it can be difficult to implement. You may need support and encouragement to get through the first few nights and days. For some people, it is helpful to keep in daily phone contact with a behavior therapist who can encourage them to stick to the program.

WHAT ABOUT READING OR WATCHING TV IN BED?

You have just learned that people with conditioned insomnia can use the stimulus-control method to unlearn the association between their bed and frustrated wakefulness. This method prohibits reading or watching television in bed. However, reading or watching TV in bed can be a good idea for people who don't experience conditioned insomnia. Many good sleepers have learned to associate reading or watching TV in bed with falling asleep.

If you have conditioned insomnia, follow the stimulus control procedures and use your bed only for sleeping. After you have broken the pattern of conditioned insomnia and learned to associate the bed with drowsiness and sleep, you may be able to resume reading or watching TV in bed. For more on this issue look at Chapter 15.

Part IV
Sleep Right in Five Nights

IT IS TIME NOW TO STEP BACK AND ASK YOURSELF WHAT YOU have learned about your sleep problem and possible solutions for it. If you recognized in Part III one or more causes of your insomnia and have undertaken the recommended solutions, you're probably sleeping better already. But you will benefit further from reading Part IV. The techniques its chapters present will improve the quality of your sleep even more.

If you *didn't* recognize in Part III a cause of your insomnia, these chapters will help you. The techniques you'll learn have proved successful with many insomnia sufferers, regardless of the origin of their particular sleep problems. A large body of research has shown that certain behavioral techniques can help induce sleep. These techniques — based on research at universities and sleep disorders centers around the world — are known also as *sleep hygiene.*

The methods can be used by adolescents or by adults of any age. Using the techniques of sleep hygiene will help you provide yourself with an ideal set of sleep circumstances. If you apply these techniques, your sleep will begin to improve noticeably in just five nights.

Chapter 13 goes over different factors related to your bed and bedroom that affect sleep. Personal preference is important in setting up an ideal sleep environment.

Chapter 14 presents several simple steps you can take during the day and evening to help yourself feel more drowsy at bedtime. These proven techniques involve diet, exercise, evening activities, bedtime routines, and an alternative to worrying in bed.

Chapter 15 tells you what to do after you climb into bed. You learn ways to relax your body, clear unwanted thoughts from your mind, and create sleep-inducing mental images.

Chapter 16 describes the Sleep CURE. This program, which is based on the techniques of sleep restriction, can help you fall asleep faster, sleep more deeply, and experience fewer nighttime awakenings.

13

Set Up Your Bedroom to Induce Sleep

DIFFERENT FACTORS IN A BEDROOM INFLUENCE HOW WELL people sleep. However, there are no firm rules for setting up a good sleep environment. People vary widely in their reactions to, and their preferences for, sleep-related bedroom conditions. For example, a ticking clock irritates some people, while others find that its monotonous sound encourages sleep. When you go through all the factors below, consider your personal preferences. Use common sense, and experiment to see which variations encourage sleep for you.

SHOULD YOU SLEEP WITH YOUR LOVED ONE?

Some people feel lonely and insecure when they sleep apart from their loved ones, and this can cause sleep to worsen. However, research shows that married couples get less deep sleep together in double beds than in separate beds.

A typical sleeper makes at least eight to twelve major posture shifts a night. When one bed partner shifts position, the other partner often moves within twenty seconds. This can be a problem, because it takes about ten minutes of undisturbed sleeping to reach the deepest level of sleep. If one person moves and disturbs the other during those ten minutes, the process of reaching deep sleep is interrupted and must begin again.

None of this means you should switch to separate beds. Most couples enjoy the physical closeness and emotional intimacy of sleeping together. Even if you have severe insomnia, you can continue to sleep with your loved one. However, a bed arrangement different from your present one might improve your sleep:

1. Buy a bigger bed. The larger the bed, the more room there is for each sleeper. A twin bed is thirty-nine inches wide and seventy-five or eighty inches long. A double bed is fifty-four by seventy-five or eighty inches. A queen is sixty by eighty inches. A king is seventy-six by eighty inches, and a California king is seventy-two by eighty-four inches.
2. Try one box spring with two half-size mattresses.
3. Place two twin beds side by side.

Either of these alternatives will reduce disturbance from your bed partner's movements during the night.

There is one situation in which you may need separate bedrooms. If your bed partner's loud snoring disturbs your sleep, first look at the section on snoring (page 59) to see what can be done to lessen the problem. If those methods don't help, you may need to consider moving to another room to get the sleep you need.

THE BED YOU SLEEP IN

In a wide-scale survey, 7 percent of American adults with sleeping problems reported that uncomfortable mattresses contributed to their sleeplessness.

Most orthopedic specialists recommend sleeping on a firm mattress and box spring. If your mattress is uncomfortable, or if it is lumpy or sags, it may be time to buy a new one. A new mattress should be turned over and rotated end to end once a month for the first six months and twice a year after that.

As with most factors regarding your sleeping environment, personal preference is important in choosing a bed. For example, a water bed nauseates some people, while others find it soothing. Some women report that water beds help them get more comfortable during pregnancy. If you choose to sleep on a water bed, it's probably best to get the "waveless" kind.

YOUR BEDDING

Cotton sheets and blankets are preferable to synthetic ones, because they create less static electricity and absorb moisture better. Some people feel most comfortable on silk sheets.

Research suggests that blue, green, and such neutral colors as beige are more soothing than red. Probably it is more important that your bedding be clean and fresh than that it be a certain color.

A mattress pad of sheep's wool has been shown to decrease movements during sleep and improve the sleep of people with arthritis. Some people without arthritis say that a woolen mattress pad is cushiony and comfortable.

Some people prefer feather or down pillows, because they conform to the shape of the head and neck more closely than foam pillows.

NOISE

Loud noise causes difficulty falling asleep, awakenings during sleep, and shallower sleep. A study in Los Angeles showed that people who lived close to the airport got on average forty-five minutes less sleep per night and less deep sleep than people who lived farther away.

A similar study in London, England, drew similar conclusions. It uncovered an additional finding that is interesting and useful. People who said they felt angry about aircraft noise were much more likely to be disturbed by the noise. This finding is an instance of how negative thoughts and self-talk can make us feel anxious or angry.

If you feel irritated or annoyed by noises at night, review the information on anger and anxiety in Chapter 10. Try to substitute calming self-talk for your angry, arousing thoughts. Below are examples of thoughts that will lead to angry sleeplessness, along with more positive and calming alternatives:

ANGRY THOUGHTS ABOUT NOISE	CORRESPONDING CALM THOUGHTS ABOUT NOISE
"The hallways and traffic here are so noisy at night!"	"It's a loud neighborhood, and the walls are really thin in these apartments. But I can get used to a little noise."
"Why do the neighbors play loud music this late?"	"This is just one night. If they start partying every night, I'll ask them to turn the volume down after ten o'clock. For tonight I'll switch on a fan to cover up the noise."
"I hate those low-flying planes!"	"I'll focus on some music instead."

Individual differences are important. Research has documented that different people have different thresholds of awakening, varying from a whisper (fifteen decibels) to a disco (one hundred decibels). Women appear more sensitive than men to noise. And the meaning of sounds makes a difference: We are more likely to be awakened by a whimpering baby or a knock on the door than by a thunderstorm.

The older we are, the more we are apt to be roused from sleep by noise. This is because older people sleep more shallowly, and less noise is required to awaken a person in shallow sleep than deep.

If your bedroom isn't quiet at night, look at where the noise comes from and what you can do to minimize it. If your apartment neighbors are loud at night, consider asking them to limit the noise adjacent to your bedroom after a reasonable hour. But not all people comply for long with such requests. There are several other ways to cope with loud neighbors as well as noise from traffic, airplanes, and barking dogs.

Certain types of draperies are designed to reduce not only light but also noise. A rug or carpet on the floor can help muffle outside sounds. Earplugs are effective for some people, although others do not like the near-total silence or the feel of them in their ears. If you use earplugs, choose a type made of soft, malleable wax that can be molded to cover the outer part of the ear.

Many people find low-frequency sounds that are steady and monotonous to be soothing and sleep-inducing. This kind of sound, called *white noise*, blends with and masks outside sounds. You can purchase a white-noise machine through specialty shops or mail-order catalogs. Some of these devices allow you to choose simulated sounds of surf, rain, or wind. You can produce your own white noise simply by running a fan, a vaporizer, or an FM radio tuned between two stations. (Incidentally, white noise can help if you want to fall asleep on an airplane. Just focus on the sound of the engines and the air whooshing outside along the fuselage.)

Listening to quiet music can also prevent you from focusing on undesired sounds. Chapter 15 includes ideas about the kinds of soothing music and environmental sounds that can encourage sleep.

INTRUDING LIGHT

Although closing your eyes keeps out most light, some finds its way through your eyelids. Dark blinds or heavy draperies will reduce the light from windows. If your bedside clock is too bright, try one with adjustable illumination. Some people wear a sleeping mask, although others can't get used to having one against their face.

Once again, let personal preference guide you. Many people find a little light comforting, as well as helpful when they get up during the night.

YOUR BEDROOM CLOCK

Many insomnia sufferers watch their bedside clocks throughout the night. They glance anxiously at them as they are trying to fall asleep, to see how long falling asleep is taking. When they awaken during the night, they check to see how much time remains before morning.

In the chapter on Sunday-night insomnia, you learned that it is important to wake up and get up at the same time each day. To do that, you need some kind of alarm clock in the bedroom. But for some people the clock should be heard and not seen. If seeing your clock makes you anxious, consider putting it across the room, under your bed, or in the top dresser drawer.

Regardless of the time of night, when you are in bed with the light off, it is time to relax and sleep. For most people a time-free environment is conducive to sleep. However, others find a bedside clock reassuring: They may think they have been awake all night, but the clock shows that in fact they have slept for several hours. Do what works best for you. If the bedroom clock makes you anxious, put it out of view. If it doesn't bother you, keep it in sight.

There is one final consideration about your bedroom clock. Some people find themselves compelled to glance at their clocks again and again, to check that the alarm is set. This behavior is among the most common manifestations of obsessive compulsive disorder, an anxiety problem described in Chapter 10. This disorder persistently affects about one person in forty. However, a larger number than that seem to have occasional difficulty with obsessive or compulsive behavior, particularly in anxious situations, such as a sleepless night before an important day.

If you find that you feel compelled to check and recheck your alarm, try this simple, effective approach. Each evening allow yourself to check the alarm *one time* and no more. When you again feel that you must look at or touch the alarm, resist the urge. You will feel anxious at first, but eventually the anxiety will wane. If you feel anxious for more than a few minutes, get out of bed, leave the bedroom, and do something else until your anxiety diminishes. Then return to bed. This time don't check the alarm, because you already have. Your anxiety will probably be less intense than before, but if you continue feeling anxious about your alarm, leave the bedroom again.

Repeat this process until you can climb into bed without rechecking the alarm. After you have broken the pattern, the next nights will be progressively easier.

ROOM TEMPERATURE AND THE AIR YOU BREATHE

Individual preferences are important when choosing room temperature. For many people the ideal temperature for sound sleep is between sixty-four and seventy degrees. Some people prefer a colder room and heavy blankets. A room temperature above seventy-five degrees causes nighttime awakening, increased movements in bed, and shallower sleep.

During the winter months, artificial heat can cause inside air to become very dry. Air that is too dry can make your nose stuffed up and your throat scratchy. A humidifier may improve your breathing and consequently help you sleep better. But air that is too humid can make you feel sweaty and clammy. Experiment to determine what works best for you.

Although many people like fresh air during sleep, there is no evidence that outside air encourages sleep better than inside air. Mark Twain told the story of a night when he stayed at a friend's house and couldn't fall asleep. He convinced himself that the reason for his insomnia was the poor ventilation. But the window was stuck, and he couldn't get it open. After tossing and turning in the darkness, he finally threw his shoe at the window in a fit of anger. He heard glass shattering, breathed in deeply, then fell asleep and slept well. The next morning he found that he had shattered not the window but rather the front of a glass-enclosed bookcase.

In this instance, Twain's action apparently helped him sleep for two reasons. First, he believed that he had removed an irritating source of frustration. Second, he believed he was now breathing the fresh air that would make sleep come more easily. These two thoughts likely helped him relax, thereby allowing sleep to overcome him.

_14_

How to Prepare for Bedtime

THIS CHAPTER PRESENTS ELEVEN GUIDELINES THAT WILL HELP you prepare your body and mind to sleep soundly. As we saw in the last chapter, making a bedroom compatible with sleep depends largely on individual preferences. However, the guidelines below should be followed by everyone.

MANAGE YOUR STRESS, ANXIETY, AND DEPRESSION

Remember that self-tests measuring these three factors are in Chapters 9 and 10. If stress, anxiety, or depression may be interfering with your sleep, review those chapters. Make a commitment to follow procedures that will help you manage these problems.

LIMIT YOUR USE OF ALCOHOL, CAFFEINE, AND TOBACCO

Chapter 8 shows how these three substances interfere with sleep. Remember, caffeine and tobacco are stimulants.

Try to avoid them from lunch until bedtime. At the very least, eliminate them for six hours before you go to bed.

Don't use booze to help you snooze. Alcohol's sedative effects may help you relax and fall asleep more easily. But your sleep will be fitful with frequent awakenings, and it will be shallow and unrestorative. Avoid alcohol for at least two hours before bedtime. If you enjoy a drink with dinner, limit it to one glass of wine or its equivalent in alcohol content.

MAINTAIN A REGULAR SLEEP-WAKE SCHEDULE

Keeping a regular sleep-wake rhythm fosters sound sleep. Getting up at the same time each day, even on weekends, is the most effective action you can take to stabilize your sleep-wake rhythm.

Some sleep experts recommend going to bed only when you are sleepy. Others advise going to bed at the same time each night. Do what feels right and what makes sense to you.

If you choose to aim for a regular bedtime, be flexible. On those nights when you feel wide-awake at your regular bedtime, don't go to bed just to lie there tossing and turning. Instead, stay up until you feel ready to sleep. But be sure to get up at your regular time the next morning.

The time you get up in the morning governs the time you will feel sleepy that night. If you arise each day at a regular time, your sleep-wake rhythm gradually will regulate itself, and you will tend to feel drowsy at the same time each night.

Some self-help books on insomnia recommend that you never go to bed until you feel sleepy. And you may recall that this was a key part of the procedure for overcoming conditioned insomnia. If you experience anxiety associated with your bed and bedroom, follow the stimulus-control procedures in Chapter 12: Don't go to bed until you feel sleepy. Then, after you have overcome your conditioned insomnia, you can begin to set up a regular bedtime.

If you don't suffer from conditioned insomnia, the best approach is to maintain a regular bedtime, to keep your circadian rhythms in sync with the twenty-four-hour day.

NAP IN THE AFTERNOON ONLY IF IT DOESN'T INTERFERE WITH YOUR NIGHTTIME SLEEP

Four out of five insomnia sufferers sleep better at night by avoiding daytime naps. There are two reasons why naps can be harmful to nighttime sleep. First, napping further disrupts sleep-wake rhythms that for insomniacs tend to be unstable and irregular. Second, an afternoon nap can diminish your body's sleep appetite and prevent the bedtime drowsiness that leads to rapid sleep onset and sound sleep.

Despite these drawbacks, 20 percent of insomnia sufferers sleep better at night when they nap during the day. These people seem to feel less anxious about going to bed at night if they know they have had a nap that day or can count on a nap the following day. This lowered anxiety level helps them relax at night and improves the quality of their sleep.

If you currently are napping on a regular or a sporadic basis, try going without a nap for a week. If you sleep better at night during this period, it's time to stop napping.

Alternatively, if you want to continue napping or experiment to see whether naps work for you, it is important to know a few facts about the napping process.

In Chapter 11 we saw that our daily circadian rhythms determine the times when we are alert and when we are sleepy. Peaks and valleys occur within the overall up-and-down patterns of our cycles. Most of us reach two daily peaks of alertness: within a few hours after waking up and during the early evening. Conversely, our level of arousal is low after midnight and during midafternoon. When we were preschool children, our afternoon slumps in alertness were more pronounced, and that was when we became sleepy and napped. Midafternoon is also the period when we as adults can nap most naturally. However, even if we don't nap, afternoon drowsiness dissipates by evening.

A midday rest or sleep period has long been an integral part of the daily routine in many cultures around the world, from India to Kenya to Greece to Mexico. It is growing less common as societies industrialize. Napping is far from universal in North American and European societies. However, many people whose circumstances permit napping use afternoon naps to restore their energy and alertness. These include children, retired people, and college students. About half of all college students nap at least once a week.

The sleep patterns of naps differ according to when in the day they occur. Morning naps resemble the REM-filled sequence at the end of a night's sleep, and we often recall vivid dreams afterward. In contrast, late-afternoon naps resemble the deep sleep at the beginning of the night, and they tend to leave us feeling groggy. Research shows that some people recover quickly from postnap grogginess, but others stay groggy for hours. For them, the recuperative value of napping is not worth the long recovery period afterward.

There are three things to avoid when you nap. First, don't nap for more than about an hour. A longer nap is more likely to interfere with nighttime sleep. Research suggests that a one-hour nap (and possibly even a shorter one) is just as refreshing as a two-hour nap. Experiment to find out what length works best for you.

Second, to minimize the nap's interference with nighttime sleep, don't nap too late in the day. If you nap after about 4:00 P.M., you are likely to descend rapidly into the deep sleep of stage 3 or 4. In Chapter 1 we found that you need only about one hour of deep sleep each twenty-four hours, and that most of your deep sleep comes in the first two hours of sleeping. A late nap cuts into your daily quota of deep sleep and diminishes your sleep appetite. This makes it harder to fall asleep at bedtime. (You may want this effect if you have to stay up late and be alert that night. In fact, it is an effective strategy to use "prophylactic napping" on the day before you'll be getting a short night's sleep. This keeps your body refreshed and your sleep rhythms on schedule.)

Third, don't nap on sporadic occasions to make up for sleep you lost the night before. "Replacement napping" will keep your sleep-wake cycle from getting into a regular rhythm. Instead, when you have a bad night, just tough it out through the next day. As discussed in Chapters 1 and 16, losing sleep won't hurt your health or your performance.

EXPOSE YOURSELF TO SUNLIGHT DURING THE DAY

Nine out of ten blind people report sleep problems: These usually include trouble falling asleep, frequent awakenings during the night, and excessive sleepiness during the day. Most blind people have these sleep problems because they have an inability to use light cues to reset their circadian clocks. For them, light cannot move through the retinohypothalamic tract from the eyes to the brain's inner clock.

Among sighted people, sleep problems are also disproportionately common for those who spend most of their time indoors. They often have insomnia for the same reason that blind people do: They receive inadequate light exposure. As Chapter 11 shows, sunlight is a powerful cue, or zeitgeber, that sets your inner circadian clock and makes its rhythm more regular. A strong circadian rhythm helps you sleep more soundly at night.

To take advantage of sunlight's effect on your sleep-wake cycle, get outside during the day as often and for as long as you can. On your lunch hour and at breaks, try to go outdoors at least for a short while. If you can't spend

much time outside during the day, avoid wearing sunglasses, so you receive a stronger light stimulus. (Check
with your doctor first, if you have eye problems and may
need sunglasses to reduce ultraviolet rays.)

You don't need to expose your skin directly to the sun.
Even on a cloudy day, if you are outside you will receive
enough light to provide alertness cues to your internal
clock. Daytime sunlight is the *yang* that fosters the *yin* of
nighttime sleep.

EXERCISE IN THE LATE AFTERNOON OR EARLY EVENING

Vigorous exercise releases excess physical energy and
mental tension. In addition, exercise directly improves
sleep in two ways: It helps you fall asleep more easily, and
it deepens your sleep.

We have seen that aerobic exercise raises the body temperature, causing a subsequent compensatory temperature
drop and consequently an improved ability to sleep four
to six hours later. To take advantage of this fact, get some
exercise during the late afternoon or early evening. If you
are used to drinking caffeine to ward off drowsiness at that
time, exercise can serve as a substitute to give you a lift.

Exercise earlier in the day is not as beneficial to sleep as
exercise during the late afternoon or early evening. If you
do aerobic exercise shortly before bedtime, your body temperature will still be elevated when you go to bed, making
it difficult to fall asleep.

To improve your sleep, it is ideal to exercise daily for
twenty to thirty minutes, hard enough to make yourself
breathe heavily. Exercising every other day is better than
not exercising at all. Research shows, though, that daily
exercisers get less deep sleep on nights when they skip
their customary exercise sessions.

Brisk walking with your arms swinging up and down is
one aerobic exercise easy to fit into most situations. For

other ideas, see the information on aerobic exercise on page 153.

Here's a lazy way to get the same sleep benefit you get from exercise: Soak in a hot bath or hot tub. Remember that the major sleep benefit of aerobic exercise is to increase your body temperature, causing a later temperature drop that facilitates sleep. On days when you can't get active exercise, you can trick your temperature system by passively heating your body. Staying in a hot tub or hot bath for twenty to thirty minutes will raise your body temperature and cause a later compensatory temperature drop. The bath has to be very hot — at least 102 degrees — so you may need to add more hot water every few minutes.

After passive body heating the subsequent drop in body temperature occurs just two to four hours later. That means you should soak in hot water two to four hours before bedtime. Some people, though, say that they sleep well right after a hot bath; probably the warmth leads to relaxation that helps them sleep despite their still-high body temperatures.

Don't neglect exercise and rely entirely on hot baths. As we have seen, aerobic exercise not only improves cardiovascular fitness and physical health. It also counteracts depression, stress, and anxiety and brings about a sense of well-being.

WIND DOWN DURING THE EVENING

Research has confirmed the commonsense notion that stressful experiences during the evening disturb nighttime sleep. Begin preparing for sleep long before your bedtime. Think of the evening as a transition period between the day's wakefulness and the night's sleep. Use this time to put aside today's troubles and tomorrow's challenges.

Make an effort to leave your work at the office. If you must bring work home, get it done early in the evening so you have time to relax before bedtime. Plan your next day's schedule and choose your next day's work clothes early in the evening, or wait until the morning.

Get household chores, family arguments, and other stressors out of the way as early in the day as possible. Most of us are touchier and less able to cope with problems late at night, so leave family problems until the next day or the weekend. Reserve the last part of the evening for enjoying a hobby, reading for pleasure, watching TV, or spending quality time with your family. Do whatever you enjoy that helps you unwind.

IF YOU TEND TO WORRY IN BED, SET UP AN ALTERNATE WORRY TIME

Sometimes you may find yourself lying in bed and ruminating about a situation at work or a personal problem. One idea leads to another, until the thoughts spin around in your mind, out of control. You rehash the situation but never find a solution. This can occur at bedtime or after awakening during the night. If you tend to worry in bed, there is a way to break the habit.

Schedule a daily period of from five minutes to a half hour for worrying. Set it up long before you go to bed: early in the evening or even earlier in the day if possible. Go into a quiet room for your worry time. But don't use your bedroom, or you may associate worries with your bedroom and develop conditioned insomnia (Chapter 12).

Use a set of three- by five-inch file cards or a notepad, whichever you prefer. Try to think of the kinds of worries that are likely to run through your mind in bed. As they come to mind, write each one down. If you use file cards, write down each worry on a separate card.

After you have written down your worries, sort them into categories. The categories may involve your job, family, finances, or whatever seems to make sense in organizing your worries. The next step is to think about the worries in each category one at a time and to figure out what you can do to solve them. Write the solution beneath each worry.

For example, if you are worried about a problem with your boss, write down a long-term plan and a step you will take to begin addressing the problem the next day. If you are worried about keeping track of everything you have to do the next day, write out a list of projects and a schedule to get them done. If you are worried about crime in your neighborhood, write yourself a note to call a locksmith or a home security company for bids on having safer door and window locks or a burglar-alarm system installed. If you are worried about getting through the month until your next paycheck, write out a list of bills and expenses, along with a plan for budgeting your money to pay them.

After you have written down your worries and solutions, put away the list or cards to review the next morning. If one of the worries surfaces while you are in bed, you can put it out of your mind because you have already dealt with it and planned a solution.

For unanticipated worries that come to you in the night, keep a card or paper near your bed. Write down the worry and work on a solution in the morning or right at the time. Some people find it is best to get up and write it down in another room, to avoid associating anxiety with the bedroom. Do whatever works for you.

Scheduling a regular time to worry gets your worries out of the way when you are thinking clearly enough to deal with them, before bedtime. Writing down a worry and its solution is a process with authority and finality that keeps the worry from continuing to run around in your mind. Your solution for each worry is a written contract with yourself to solve the problem or to cope with it however you can.

You may want to schedule a worry time every evening. If no worries come or if you need only a few minutes to deal with them, get up gratefully and continue on with your evening. As an alternative, you can set up worry times only when things seem particularly troublesome.

USE NUTRITION TO HELP YOU SLEEP

At bedtime your stomach should be neither too full nor too empty. The discomfort of a full stomach can interfere with sleep, while hunger can make it harder to fall asleep and can awaken you during the night.

Try eating a light bedtime snack with calories saved from earlier in the day. A combination of carbohydrates and protein, such as cheese and crackers or cereal and milk, seems to have a mild sleep-inducing effect for some people. This effect appears to be due in part to the action of digestive hormones and in part to natural *tryptophan* in the food.

TRYPTOPHAN

Tryptophan is a naturally occurring amino acid found in such protein-rich foods as milk, cheese, eggs, beans, meat, and poultry. The average person consumes one to two grams of tryptophan daily. The body converts tryptophan to the brain chemical *serotonin,* which slows down nerve activity. Research shows that tryptophan helps about half of all insomnia sufferers, including those in both major categories: trouble falling asleep and trouble staying asleep. The sleep-inducing effects of tryptophan are mild, even for those people it helps.

Synthetic tryptophan was once available without a prescription. However, in 1989 it was taken off the market because of various side effects, including aching muscles and joints, fatigue, skin rash, and blood disorders. These adverse effects seem to be due not to the amino acid itself but rather to contaminants used in manufacturing it.

If synthetic tryptophan again becomes available in prescription or nonprescription form, discuss with your doctor whether you should try it.

VITAMINS, MINERALS, HERBS

Certain types of vitamins, minerals, and herbs help some people to sleep better. As with tryptophan, sleep effects from these substances typically are mild and vary greatly from person to person. Allow one week to pass before expecting results, to give your body time to make adjustments.

Taking 50 to 100 mg of vitamin B$_3$, also called *niacin*, improves some cases of insomnia that accompany mild depression. Vitamin B$_{12}$ and another B vitamin, *folic acid*, seem to help some people sleep better. You can buy B complex multivitamin supplements: B-50 products provide 50 mg of each of the B vitamins, and B-100 products provide 100 mg of each. Taking one a day of either supplement may be helpful.

Some people experience sleeplessness from taking the B vitamins. For this reason, if you use them, it is important to monitor your particular reaction.

The minerals *magnesium* and *calcium* are natural sedatives that help some people relax and sleep better. Because these minerals are depleted rapidly from the body during stress reactions, deficiencies occur when they are needed most. Some experts recommend taking magnesium and calcium in a one-to-one ratio, about one gram of each mineral. Other authorities recommend taking them in a one-to-two ratio, about 500 mg of magnesium and one gram of calcium. Some tablets combine the two minerals for convenience.

Valerian, from the root of a European plant, is an herb with sedating properties. It was the major sedative used in the Western industrialized world before barbiturate drugs were invented in the early part of this century. In Europe, valerian still is used widely as a relaxant. One gram shortly before bedtime is the usual recommended dose. Valerian can be taken in tincture or tablet form, or it can be brewed as a tea.

A few people are sensitive to valerian and experience a kind of hangover effect the next morning after a one-gram dose; for them, a much smaller dose may improve sleep with no hangover. Again, it is important to monitor your reaction to different substances.

FOODS TO AVOID

At dinner and during the evening, stay away from fats and from any foods that are heavily spiced, especially with garlic. These foods can give you indigestion or heartburn that interferes with sleep. People who are sensitive to monosodium glutamate (MSG) can suffer insomnia from stimulant effects of this food additive. Be aware that MSG is often used in meat tenderizers and Chinese food. If MSG disrupts your sleep, be sure it's not added to the food you eat.

THINK POSITIVELY ABOUT SLEEP AND ABOUT THE STEPS YOU CAN TAKE TO IMPROVE YOUR SLEEP

In Chapters 9 and 10 we saw how our thoughts affect our feelings. We also learned how to identify negative thoughts and substitute positive thoughts for them. Use these techniques. If you find yourself forming thoughts like one of those on the left side of the following chart, interrupt yourself and substitute the corresponding thought on the right:

NEGATIVE THOUGHTS THAT DISRUPT SLEEP	*POSITIVE THOUGHTS THAT PROMOTE SLEEP*
"I bet I'll lie awake again tonight."	"I'm going to limit coffee today and exercise hard after work. Those steps will help me sleep tonight."

"Why does my spouse sleep better than I do? It's not fair!"	"Some people naturally sleep better than others. But if I keep up with my sleep hygiene, I'll be sleeping better and better."
"What if I can't sleep again tonight?"	"Sleep will come when I need it."

USE A BEDTIME ROUTINE TO FOSTER SLEEP

Most parents recognize the importance of giving young children a nightly routine to help them prepare for sleep. This may involve such activities as brushing teeth, taking a bath, putting on pajamas, and hearing a lullaby.

The sound behavioral and commonsense principle of a bedtime routine is helpful for adults as well as for children. A regularly repeated routine can affect thoughts, emotions, and the body's level of arousal. It carries a special meaning because of its association with another dimension of our life — in this case, with sleep.

A bedtime routine can help you gradually break your ties with daytime details and problems. As you prepare for bed, try to shift your attention from thinking about the past and future to experiencing the present moment. A bedtime routine has the most effect if you are conscious of your actions as you perform them, rather than thinking about other things.

Good sleepers become more relaxed and drowsy as they walk the dog, turn out the lights, check on the children, brush their teeth, put on their nightclothes, and go through the rest of their nightly bedtime routine.

Not all bedtime routines are relaxing, however. Such activities as choosing clothes to wear to work, planning a schedule, and organizing papers for tomorrow's work day can be mentally arousing rather than soothing. Let personal preferences guide you. Watching the late-night news is a pleasant quasi-social event for some people, but it tends to be upsetting for others. Setting an alarm clock makes some people anxious. We have seen that you should get up at the same time each morning, so you may not need to reset your alarm each night.

Saying good night to a loved one is a particularly reassuring part of a bedtime routine. If you live alone, you still can say good night to your room as you switch off the light. Say good night to your pet, your favorite picture, a musical instrument, whatever is important to you. This routine can take on a ritual quality, eliciting associations with past experiences of family living or memories of being loved.

_15_

What to Do in Bed

THIS CHAPTER PRESENTS EIGHT GUIDELINES FOR WHAT TO DO after you climb into bed. These can help induce sleep by making your body and mind more relaxed and receptive to sleep. You can use these procedures in two situations: to fall asleep when you first go to bed and to return to sleep after a nighttime awakening.

Think of these as last resorts. By themselves they will not solve a sleep problem. You can't keep irregular hours, let stress build uncontrolled to high levels, avoid exercise, and indulge in alcohol or caffeine late in the day, then expect to fall asleep easily by using bedtime techniques. What you learn here will be effective only as a complement to the other methods of sleep hygiene presented in the last two chapters.

DON'T LET FEAR OF INSOMNIA KEEP YOU AWAKE

Anxiety about the possibility of insomnia often causes lost sleep. The more you worry about sleep, the worse you will sleep. However, there is no reason to fear insomnia. This may be hard to believe at 2:00 A.M., when you are lying in bed afraid that your insomnia will keep you from being at your best for an important event during the day. But a large body of research shows that sleep loss will not hurt your performance the next day.

Often we sleep most poorly the night before an important event. Some astronauts have said that they had a hard time falling asleep the night before a launch. Olympic athletes generally are excellent sleepers, with only 3 percent reporting significant insomnia and 10 percent reporting occasional insomnia. However, on nights before international competitions they lose an average of one to three hours of sleep. It can be reassuring to know that you are not the only one who wrestles with insomnia the night before a big day.

It is even more reassuring to know the facts about sleep loss and performance. If you sometimes worry about sleeplessness, review the section in Chapter 1 (page 31) about the consequences of losing sleep. Sleep loss leads to no physical or mental health problems, in the short term or the long run.

During active or important events, your body's surge of adrenaline will overcome any effects of sleep loss. According to research conducted in France, people secrete more adrenaline after being sleep-deprived than after being well rested. So the day after a poor night's sleep you will "get your juices flowing" to compensate for sleep loss. For example, Olympic athletes experience no adverse effects on their performances when they lose sleep the night before a competitive event. Even if you don't sleep at all, your performance won't suffer when you catch an early flight, deliver a speech, take an exam, or run a race.

If you find yourself lying in bed worrying about losing sleep, interrupt the thoughts and substitute more positive ones. For example, if you are thinking, "I'll be worthless at the meeting tomorrow if I don't fall asleep soon," substitute the thought "Even if I don't sleep much tonight, I'll do fine at work tomorrow."

READ OR WATCH TV IN BED IF IT HELPS YOU RELAX AND FALL ASLEEP; IF IT STIMULATES YOU, DO IT IN ANOTHER ROOM

Many people enjoy reading, watching TV, or listening to quiet music in bed. These pastimes can help induce sleep because they are somewhat passive mentally and require no effort physically. Before you know it, sleep just might sneak in by the back door as you are lying in bed.

If reading always leads to sleep, over time sleep will become a conditioned response to reading. Eventually you will associate reading in bed with falling asleep, so that the stimulus of reading in bed helps elicit the sleep response. This connection is equally true for watching TV or listening to music.

Lying in bed comfortably reading, watching TV, or listening to music is more restful than tossing and turning. Even if you are awake much of the night, you will get more rest and feel less frustrated than if you had been tossing and turning, trying to fall sleep.

If you find that you fall asleep while reading, watching TV, or listening to music, consider making two bedroom investments. First, buy a timer so your bedside lamp will switch off on its own. Second, buy a TV with a remote control and sleep timer, or buy a radio with a cassette or compact disc player and a sleep timer. A sleep timer is useful because even if music or TV helps you relax and fall asleep, continuing sounds can prevent you from reaching the deepest levels of sleep. Consider these investments worthwhile if they improve your sleep; after all, you spend a third of your life sleeping.

Use common sense in choosing what to see, hear, or read in bed. If you have a TV in your bedroom, you may want to add a VCR so that you can watch a program likely to help you relax. A TV show with action or suspense may stimulate you and keep you from falling asleep. A talk show, drama, or documentary works better for some people. Others enjoy a light nightly rerun (for example, the programs *M*A*S*H* or *Cheers*) after the late news. Whatever you prefer, keep the TV volume and brightness controls down low.

Select reading material that seems to help you relax. Many people find that fiction allows them to enter a new world. Nonfiction can have the same effect. For most people it's best to avoid reading job-related material at bedtime, because it can elicit stressful associations related to work.

If you enjoy music in bed, there are more choices than an easy-listening radio station. Consider nonsymphonic classical music by soloists and small chamber groups. Certain types of jazz are melodious and soothing. Some forms of New Age music are intended to promote calm.

International or folk music can be at once interesting and restful. Music in a different language, like instrumental music, will not distract you with the meaning of its words. International and folk music seem somehow to provide a tie to the six billion other inhabitants of the Earth — about two billion of whom are sleeping now. This feeling of a bond with the rest of humanity helps some people relax and fall asleep.

It can be a soothing and pleasant experience to fall asleep to recorded environmental sounds. These include ocean surf, a rainstorm, a tropical forest, and dusk on a woodland pond. Environmental sounds are available on tape and compact disc at some music stores and bookstores.

You may have noticed that this guideline — to consider reading or watching TV in bed — contradicts the stimulus-control procedures for unlearning conditioned insomnia that we saw earlier. In the stimulus-control method, the person is to use the bed only for sleeping. Stimulus control is designed to help unlearn a conditioned fear of sleep and the sleep environment. If you have come to associate your bed and bedroom with anxiety and frustrated sleeplessness rather than drowsiness, you should review the information in Chapter 12 and use the bed only for sleeping. Otherwise, it may be helpful to read or watch TV in bed.

DON'T TRY TO SLEEP; INSTEAD LIE PASSIVELY IN BED AND ALLOW SLEEP TO OVERCOME YOU

You can't achieve sleep by an act of will. The more you try to fall asleep, the more you will become anxious, physiologically aroused, and afraid of insomnia. Veteran University of Florida researcher Dr. Wilse Webb wrote in *Sleep: The Gentle Tyrant* (Boulton, Mass.: Anker Publishing, 1992): "Sleep is like love or happiness. If you pursue it too ardently, it will evade you."

Sleep therapists often observe that trying to sleep leads to sleeplessness. This phenomenon also was documented experimentally in a 1985 study published in the journal *Sleep Research*. In that study, subjects who were offered twenty-five dollars if they could fall asleep quickly took about twice as long to fall asleep as subjects offered no reward.

Don't think of sleep as something you can pursue and capture. Instead, entice sleep to come to you. Think of sleep as a gentle, overpowering force that can take you as a willing captive if you let go and allow it.

Imagine sleep a wave in the ocean and yourself a surfer. If you position yourself and wait, the wave will overtake you and sweep you away.

Or think of sleep as a friend who may visit. If you make the right preparations, your friend will arrive in her own good time. And she likes to come unexpectedly.

Each of these metaphors illustrates a passive approach to falling asleep. If your body is ready for sleep and if you maintain a calm and relaxed state for ten to twenty minutes, it is likely that sleep will overcome you.

Remember, your thoughts are important. If you find yourself thinking, "Why can't I sleep?" or "I've got to fall asleep," substitute thoughts like "Sleep will come when it's time" or "If I continue to relax, I'll fall asleep before long."

MAKING LOVE CAN BE HELPFUL

Many people find that sex helps bring about physical and mental relaxation, which in turn induces sleep. It burns about 150 calories, it reaffirms your relationship with your bed partner, and it is fun.

Sex will encourage sleep if you feel loved and loving afterward. However, if it makes you feel used or frustrated, you will be unhappy or tense. In that case, sex can lead to a poor night's sleep.

LET YOUR BODY CHOOSE YOUR SLEEP POSITION

You can't easily determine the position you sleep in, because you unconsciously change position many times a night. However, you can pick the position you *fall* asleep in.

There is no right or wrong body position for falling sleep. Just let your body settle into a position that feels comfortable and natural.

The most common sleep position is lying on the side, with arms and legs bent. Side sleep positions range from almost straight to semifetal. Sleeping on the back is the next most frequent position. Sleeping on the stomach is least common.

Poor sleepers spend more sleep time on their backs than good sleepers do. But many good sleepers also sleep on their backs. Sleeping on the back is associated with poor sleep in part because that position facilitates the respiratory problems of snoring and sleep apnea. So if you snore or have apnea, avoid sleeping on your back, and read those sections in Chapters 2 and 6. Otherwise fall asleep on your back if that feels most comfortable.

Some people have problems with their necks or spines when they sleep on their stomachs. Breathing can also be difficult. But other people sleep on their stomachs and experience none of these problems. Let your body guide you.

USE SYSTEMATIC RELAXATION IF YOU FEEL PHYSICALLY TENSE

Remember from Chapter 2 that not all insomnia sufferers are physically tense. Check for yourself. Do your muscles feel tense and tight? Is your breathing fast and shallow? If you experience these indicators of physical tension, physical relaxation may help you become relaxed and more receptive to sleep. Review the section in Chapter 10 on relaxation skills, and look at the three different relaxation scripts in Appendix 1.

Don't use relaxation techniques in bed until you have become reasonably skilled by practicing them in a chair first. Otherwise, you may be unsuccessful at using relaxation in bed, and you will learn to associate the techniques with physical tension and bedtime frustration rather than with relaxation and sleep.

Abdominal breathing is an easy technique to use in bed. Tense-and-release relaxation is an excellent method for learning deep muscle relaxation. However, many people find passive relaxation better for inducing sleep in bed, because it includes no tension component.

USE MENTAL IMAGERY IF YOUR MIND IS TENSE OR YOUR THOUGHTS ARE RACING

Ancient pastoral peoples counted sheep in their minds as a way to fall asleep. This technique can be effective because it is a boring, monotonous task that occupies your mind and prevents troubling thoughts from arising long enough to permit sleep to arrive. Counting sheep is one example of *mental imagery*, or forming pictures in your mind's eye.

Mental imagery can block out troublesome thoughts that buzz in your brain, in much the same way that electronic jamming equipment blocks radio broadcasts.

Many mental-imagery techniques can help induce sleep. Here are some to consider. Go through the list below and choose one that you might feel comfortable with.

Before beginning each technique, first take a few deep, relaxing breaths from your abdomen. Let your body become limp against the bed.

- Float along. *Imagine a scene in which you are floating, surrounded and supported by a soft surface. Feel yourself lying on a billowy cloud with warm breezes all around. Or imagine yourself lying on an air mattress in a warm and gentle sea, with the waves softly lapping as they support you.*

- Drift downward to relaxation. *An image of moving downward is very relaxing to some people. Imagine yourself walking slowly down a staircase or riding down an elevator or escalator. As you go down, let yourself sink more deeply into relaxation.*

  If you choose to reach the bottom, have the elevator doors open, or step off the escalator or stairs. Passively create a pleasant, relaxing place. After a while there, you can go down a conveyance to a deeper level of relaxation if you want. Use your imagination, and be creative in devising restful places in your mind.

- Count down to relaxation. *Count down very slowly, beginning with one hundred. Visualize each number, and when you come to each, release more tension and relax more deeply. Visualize the numbers in a downward progression, with each one standing on a staircase one step lower than the previous one. If you like, make it a winding marble staircase with a beautiful brass banister.*

  As a variation, think of a deep velvety blackboard, com-

pletely clean. *Slowly write the number "100." Then slowly erase it, and write "99." Erase that, and write "98," and so on.*

You can abbreviate this technique by counting down from ten to one or from five to one.

Be a hero. *In the book* Everybody's Guide to Natural Sleep *by Philip Goldberg and Daniel Kaufman (Los Angeles: Jeremy P. Tarcher, Inc., 1990), a sportswriter is quoted telling of a fantasy he has fallen asleep to every night since he was ten years old:*

> *"As soon as I close my eyes, I imagine a baseball scene. It is usually the last inning of the last game of the World Series. It's two out, the score is tied, and the bases are loaded. I am either the centerfielder or the relief pitcher just brought in from the bullpen. If I'm in center field, the batter hits a tremendous fly ball that I overhaul by leaping to the top of a ten-foot fence, catching it just before the ball reaches the stands. If I'm the relief pitcher, I strike the batter out. Then, after leaving the field to the appreciative roar of the crowd, I lead off the bottom of the ninth with a game-winning home run. I usually fall asleep before I get to the locker room for the champagne party."*

Create any world where you are a hero. For example, you can walk through a park filled with hundreds of children and give a balloon to each appreciative child. You may want to imagine that your bundle of balloons is your tension, which dissipates bit by bit as you give away each balloon.

Positive emotions are conductive to falling asleep. Experiment with different fantasies, until you find one that makes you feel good.

• Take a vacation. *Enjoy an around-the-world trip in which everything goes right. Imagine the airplane or boat taking off and landing at each destination. You may want to bring along your sleeping partner or another person you love.*

• Create a peaceful scene. *Imagine a calm and restful scene in your mind. Don't just watch; try to experience yourself inside the scene. And don't just see the images; feel, hear, and smell everything in the environment.*

Appendix 2 presents a sample scene for inducing peaceful relaxation. Consider tape recording that scene or one of your own creation, so you can listen to it in bed. Lie down and enter that world in your mind.

IF YOU CAN'T SLEEP, DO SOMETHING ELSE

If you have been lying in bed restless and unable to sleep for ten or twenty minutes, don't stay there tossing and turning. That will make you feel more frustrated and tense.

Don't watch the clock to see how long it's been since you turned out the light. If you've been lying in bed awhile and you feel unable to sleep, it's time to do something else. Turn on the light and read, or get up, put on a robe and slippers, and go to another room.

Don't think of time awake at night as lost time; instead consider it newfound time that you can use. We will return to this theme in the book's next and final chapter.

16
The Sleep CURE

THE SLEEP CURE IS BASED ON THE METHOD OF SLEEP RE-striction. This strategy derives from many research studies that consistently have documented one important fact: *Reducing time in bed causes a person to fall asleep faster, sleep more deeply, and experience fewer nighttime awakenings.*

Sleep restriction as a specific behavioral treatment for insomnia was introduced in a 1983 article in the journal *Sleep Research.* This study was published by a joint research team from the Sleep Disorders Center of the City University of New York and the Sleep-Wake Disorders Center of Montefiore Medical Center in New York. Since that classic research report by Dr. Arthur Spielman and his colleagues, sleep specialists everywhere have used sleep restriction as a strategy to treat insomnia.

The Sleep CURE will help you sleep more efficiently and improve the quality of your sleep. A temporary side effect of sleep restriction is daytime sleepiness. Because of that, it takes determination to keep on with the program, and not everyone can. For example, in a major sleep-restriction research report published in 1987 in the journal *Sleep,* twelve of forty-nine subjects dropped out of the study because they couldn't tolerate daytime sleepiness. But the thirty-seven subjects who continued with the program benefited greatly from sleep restriction. Their time falling asleep dropped by an average of twenty-nine minutes. Their average time lying awake in bed decreased by one hour and forty-nine minutes. Their total sleep time increased, even though they spent less time in bed. And their initial daytime sleepiness disappeared; subjects were much less sleepy during the day at the end of sleep restriction than before they had begun the program. A nine-month follow-up showed that the subjects maintained their sleep improvement.

Early research on sleep restriction was done with young adults and middle-aged people. But this insomnia treatment also has proved effective with older adults. In a 1991 study published in the *Journal of Gerontology* by researchers from the Stanford University School of Medicine, a group of adults with an average age of sixty-seven used sleep restriction. It helped older adults on average fall asleep twenty-three minutes faster and lie awake in bed one hour and fourteen minutes less during the night.

Sleep restriction can be an effective treatment for nearly all types of insomnia. However, it is not appropriate for insomnia caused by sleep apnea (Chapter 6), delayed or advanced sleep phase syndrome (Chapter 11), or night work (Appendix 3).

After just a few nights of following this plan, you will be falling asleep more quickly and sleeping more soundly. You can easily remember the four steps of this plan by thinking of the letters in the acronym CURE.

C. Cut down on your time in bed.

U. Use your time awake at night as new-found time.

R. Relax about sleeping less, because it won't hurt your health or your performance.

E. Every day get out of bed at the same time.

Let's examine these four steps, one at a time.

CUT DOWN ON YOUR TIME IN BED

It may sound paradoxical, but if you spend less time in bed, your sleep will improve. You will fall asleep more easily, sleep more deeply, and experience fewer nighttime awakenings. As you will see, it's easy to set up a sleep-restriction plan to improve the quality of your sleep.

Many insomnia sufferers believe that they need to spend extra time in bed to make up for the poor sleep they have been getting. But going to bed early or sleeping in late will cause your sleep to be less deep and less restorative. For example, if you need seven hours of sleep but stay in bed for nine, the seven hours will tend to get spread out thinly over nine hours. Your sleep will be shallow and fragmented with frequent awakenings.

A cycle of sleeplessness can develop from spending too much time in bed. The pattern begins when you start to sleep badly because of poor sleep habits, stress, or any other reason. Because you feel fatigued, you spend more time in bed to try to catch up on sleep. Then, because you lie in bed longer than you need to, you sleep less soundly. Consequently, you spend even more time in bed, leading to shallow sleep that is even less refreshing. This self-perpetuating circle strengthens as it goes on and on.

When you lie in bed too long, the night's overall sleep will be less efficient and restorative, causing you to awaken feeling tired rather than refreshed. Psychologist Peter Hauri of the Mayo Clinic likens sleep to water. A given quantity may cover a surface, but if you spread it over a larger area, you no longer will cover the surface well. The water will be shallower, and gaps will appear between different sections of water. Similarly, spreading a night's sleep over too long a period of time will lead to sleep that is shallow and fragmented.

If you suffer from insomnia, you need to spend *less* time in bed rather than more. Reducing time in bed concentrates and solidifies your sleep into a tighter package. The amount of deep sleep actually increases. What decreases is the shallower and less restorative sleep of stages 1 and 2.

Subjects in sleep-reduction experiments sleep more efficiently than usual. They fall asleep more quickly, sleep more deeply, have fewer and shorter nighttime awakenings, and maintain sleep until it's time to awaken. These are exactly the kinds of changes insomnia sufferers seek.

To improve your sleep, you need to restrict your sleep schedule by aiming for less time in bed and less time asleep. It's easy to do. Just follow these three steps:

1. Use your sleep log to calculate your average amount of nighttime sleep — not the hours you lie in bed. Plan to stay in bed only the length of your average sleep time.

   If you choose not to complete a sleep log, you can use an alternate method to determine how long to stay in bed. Think back to a time before your sleeping problems began. Estimate how long you slept then, and plan to stay in bed only that amount of time.

   Remember, the more you cut down your time in bed, the more sound your sleep will become.

2. Choose a regular wake-up time. For most people, a job schedule determines when they wake up. If you don't have a certain hour you need to awaken, you can let personal preference guide you. In either case, stick to your chosen wake-up time seven days a week. (After you have solidified your sleep and gotten over the worst of your insomnia, you can sleep one extra hour later on weekend mornings if you want. But it's better to be consistent on weekends, too.)

3. Determine a regular bedtime. Start from your wake-up time, and subtract back the number of sleep hours you calculated in Step 1 above.

For example, if you average six hours of sleep each night — even though you may lie in bed much longer — aim initially to stay in bed for only six hours. Choose a regular wake-up time, and go to bed six hours earlier. If you plan to wake up regularly at 7:00 A.M., then you would go to bed six hours earlier, at 1:00 A.M.

At first, your body may complain because it's not used to spending less time in bed. It may take up to several weeks for your body to adjust entirely to lying down for a shorter time. You will probably feel sleepier than usual when you wake up and during the day. But stick to the new schedule, and don't nap during the day.

After a few nights, evaluate how well you are sleeping. If you find that you fall asleep sooner and sleep more soundly through the night than before, skip the next paragraph and read the one that follows it.

If you *don't* sleep well after several nights of the later bedtime — 1:00 A.M. in our example — maybe your body needs less sleep than you thought. To investigate this possibility, for the next few nights go to bed a half hour later. Instead of going to bed at 1:00 A.M., try staying up until 1:30. If that later bedtime doesn't help you fall asleep and stay asleep, stay up another half hour to 2:00 A.M.

After you begin to fall asleep and sleep well through the night regularly, you can try to increase your allotted sleep time by thirty minutes. So in our example, if you sleep well on a 1:00 A.M. to 7:00 A.M. schedule, try moving your bedtime back to 12:30 A.M. Then, if you sleep well for a few nights with this new schedule, move your bedtime back another half hour, to midnight. You'll know you're trying to sleep too long when you reach a point where you no longer fall asleep quickly and sleep well through the night.

Once you find your ideal bedtime and sleep schedule, *stay with it.* Of course, if circumstances in your life change, you may want to alter your sleep-wake schedule accordingly. For example, if you get a different job and can sleep in daily an hour later each day, feel free to do so. But be sure also to move your bedtime up an hour later, so you continue to allot the same number of hours for sleeping. Alter your sleep-wake schedule only if you intend to keep the new schedule for a prolonged period of time.

Use your time awake at night as newfound time

Try to remember when you were a child. Probably you protested when your parents made you go to bed. If you couldn't fall asleep or woke up early, it felt like a treat. You noticed the magical hush of the night. You played with your toys, read a book, or turned on the TV with the sound way down low. Nobody bothered you or told you what to do. You savored the rare middle-of-the-night opportunity for quiet privacy.

It's not so hard to recapture some of your childhood feeling of happiness when you find yourself with unexpected time alone at night. Just think how many times you've wished that you had extra time to catch up on chores or to pursue a hobby. The Sleep CURE will give you newfound time that wasn't available to you before. These are the hours when you used to lie in bed, sleeping shallowly or trying in vain to sleep.

Many people find that when they can't sleep at night, reading, watching TV, or a quiet hobby relaxes them and helps them fall asleep. However, for some severe insomnia sufferers, it's best not to read a good book or watch a good video, because enjoyable activities can reinforce late-night wakefulness and cause the pattern to persist. For them, it's better to begin some of the household chores they've been putting off: cleaning out a drawer, doing laundry, paying bills, organizing a closet. If you use your newfound time to get things done, you'll be surprised and pleased at how much you can accomplish with those hours you used to spend tossing and turning, trying to fall asleep. And working on household chores may make insomnia less rewarding.

Experiment on different nights, so you can gauge for yourself if household chores or enjoyable activities work better to help you feel drowsy when you're up late at night.

RELAX ABOUT SLEEPING LESS, BECAUSE IT WON'T HURT YOUR
HEALTH OR YOUR PERFORMANCE

Many people think that sleeping less will lead to negative health consequences and poor performance on the job. However, it is well documented that cutting down on sleep time harms neither physical nor mental health; nor does it lower daytime performance significantly. If you feel worried about the idea of sleeping less, review the section about the consequences of sleep loss in Chapter 1 (page 31).

The human body can function remarkably well under such stress as minor infections or sleep loss. When you have a cold, you manage to get through the days and get your work done without worrying about the cold or its effects on your performance. Similarly, when you sleep poorly, the best thing to do is to go about your business the next day without focusing on last night's sleep loss. You may feel a little tired and irritable, but your performance won't suffer.

Although sleep restriction may not be an ideal way of life,

it is a powerful way to overcome an insomnia problem. Then, after you have reduced or eliminated your insomnia, you can return gradually to a longer sleep schedule with the procedure outlined earlier in this chapter.

Alternatively, you can continue sleeping less. In sleep-restriction experiments, subjects are required to sleep less than their usual amount. Interestingly, after these experiments have ended, subjects typically continue sleeping one to two and a half hours less than they slept before the experiment started. This suggests that originally they were getting more sleep than they needed.

British sleep researcher Dr. James Horne of Loughborough University reviewed a large body of research on human sleep needs in his scholarly book *Why We Sleep.* (Oxford University Press, 1988). He argues that the night's first three sleep cycles — four to five hours — provide all the sleep we need. He calls this *core sleep.* The remaining three hours or so are *optional sleep,* which can be eliminated without significant consequences, because sleep toward the end of the night is shallower and less restorative than sleep earlier in the night. Horne concludes that "we probably do not really need the last few hours of a typical night's sleep, and sleep loss is far less harmful than most would think." Many sleep researchers on both sides of the Atlantic agree with Horne.

Every day get out of bed at the same time

Alexandre Dumas, the French novelist who wrote *The Three Musketeers*, had severe insomnia. He consulted his doctor, who advised him to eat an apple under the Arc de Triomphe each morning at seven o'clock. Dumas followed the recommendation and soon found that his insomnia was cured. In fact, though, neither the apple nor the place he ate it made a difference. But when he followed the regimen his wise doctor advised, he had to get out of bed at the same time each morning.

A regular waking time anchors and stabilizes your sleep-wake rhythm by resetting your internal clock to correspond to the twenty-four-hour day. Except for the crucial steps of cutting out nighttime caffeine, nicotine, and alcohol, simply waking up at the same time each day will do more to improve the quality of your sleep than any other action you can take.

So get out of bed at the same time each morning, regardless of how late you stay up at night. Don't oversleep, even if you slept very little the night before. And don't linger too long in bed after you wake up, or you may fall back asleep, destabilizing your internal rhythms.

When you follow the Sleep CURE, you may have a hard time getting out of bed the first few mornings. At first, if your body is accustomed to lying in bed a certain number of hours each night, it will resist the change to spending less time in bed. Here are some suggestions for waking yourself up in the morning to face the day:

- *Realize that you're not the only person who has a hard time dragging out of bed. Many people are slow starters in the morning. Pablo Picasso said, "I understand why they execute condemned men at dawn. I just have to see the dawn in order to have my head roll all by itself." Don't feel guilty or inferior because you don't leap out of bed ready to take on the world.*

- *Try waking up one part at a time. When your alarm goes off, don't burrow back into your pillow. Instead, bend each of your fingers one at a time. Then try your toes. Next take a deep breath. Bend one arm, then the other. Bend your legs one at a time. Move your head from side to side. Now do the hardest part: Put your feet on the floor. The worst is over. Stand up and stretch your arms over your head. You're up!*

  Alternatively, you may prefer to roll out of bed all at once. It's like entering a cold swimming pool. You can do it a little at a time, or you can just jump in. Different people have different preferences. Either way, the water will feel much better in just a few minutes.

- *Place your clock on a dresser, and set it to wake to the alarm rather than to music. That way you will have to get out of bed.*
  Again there is an alternative: You may find that waking to music or a news program is less jarring than the buzz of an alarm.

- *Expose yourself to bright light in the morning. Chapter 11 shows how bright light helps synchronize your circadian rhythms to the start of a daytime period of alertness. Many people seem to know this instinctively; they open the curtains or raise the window shades as soon as they awaken in the morning. Try to go outside into the sunlight for at least a few minutes, to receive a light stimulus signaling your brain that it is time to be alert.*

- *Do whatever works to wake yourself up. Try stretching exercises. Take a few deep breaths. Shower. A little exercise, such as a brisk walk around the block, can activate your body's alerting mechanism.*

- *Think positively about the coming day. Remember what you learned in the chapters on depression and on stress and anxiety: The thoughts you choose to think affect how you feel. Try to think about something pleasant that will happen during the day.*

If you feel drowsy during the day, do more stretching and deep breathing. Try to get in some physical exercise, even if it's just a brisk walk at lunchtime or a break. And keep busy, because activity counters drowsiness.

You can look forward to sleeping better soon. If you stick to a consistent wake-up time, within just a few days your body will demand sleep at a reasonable bedtime that will become increasingly regular.

Going to bed at the same time each night is not as critical as getting up at a regular time, but for most people it is helpful to aim for the same bedtime each night. If your sleep begins around the same predictable hour each night, your body will more easily stabilize and maintain its circadian sleep-wake cycle.

Of course, there will be occasions when you want to stay up past your usual bedtime. You don't have to adhere to a rigid bedtime schedule. Just be sure that you get out of bed at the same time every morning, even after a late night.

Sleep restriction is a simple behavioral method you can use to overcome insomnia. Go to bed late, and get up at the same time each day. If you still don't sleep well, go to bed even later. After you begin sleeping better, you can gradually go to bed earlier and sleep longer. Whenever your insomnia returns, just go to bed late again.

Cut down your time in bed.

Use your time awake at night as newfound time.

Relax about sleeping less, because it won't hurt your health or your performance.

Every day get out of bed at the same time.

That's the Sleep CURE — a sensible plan based on proven methods of sleep restriction that will help you fall asleep more quickly and sleep more soundly through the night.

Epilogue:
Maintain Good Sleep Habits over the Years

IN THIS BOOK YOU HAVE LEARNED ABOUT THE DIFFERENT kinds of sleep problems and how to diagnose your own sleeplessness. If you discovered what causes your insomnia, you have been able to take steps to address the cause or causes.

Even if you have not found the cause of your poor sleep, following the techniques in Part IV will help you fall asleep faster and sleep more soundly through the night. Knowing and practicing those methods of sleep hygiene will make a big difference in the quality of your sleep.

Knowledge is power. Use what you've learned to take charge of the night.

KEEP REALISTIC GOALS

Chapter 1 showed that different people require different amounts of sleep. Trying to get more sleep than your body needs is a sure way to manufacture an insomnia problem.

Remember what you just learned in Chapter 16 about the importance of cutting down your time in bed to the amount you need, and no more.

In Chapter 1 you also found that some people inherently sleep better than others. You may never sleep as well as your spouse, and you may never sleep soundly through the night every night. Aiming for an unrealistic goal is likely to lead to frustration. However, you can use what you've learned in this book to make the quality of your sleep as good as your genetic predisposition permits.

KEEP TRACK OF YOUR PROGRESS

It is better to prevent a problem than to solve one. And it is easier to solve a mild problem than a severe one. However, most of us do not think preventively and tend to let mild problems slide until they become severe.

If you have improved the quality of your sleep with the program in this book, don't be complacent about your progress. Keep alert to recurrences of insomnia. It is not unusual for people to improve a behavior problem, only to find that the improvements slip away when they become lax and reduce their efforts.

Make your sleep-improvement program a lifelong practice. Use the techniques you have learned until they become second nature. Make them part of your daily and nightly routines, so that you follow the practices of good sleep hygiene without concentrating on them. Think of good sleep habits the way you think of habits like brushing your teeth or combing your hair. If you make them a part of your regular routine, you won't forget to follow them.

KEEP A GOOD ATTITUDE

The things we tell ourselves make a big difference in how we feel. Remember what you learned in Chapters 9 and

10 about how self-talk can worsen stress, anxiety, and depression.

This principle applies to insomnia, too. If you repeat self-defeating statements to yourself like "I'll never get better" or "Pills are the only answer," you will come to believe them.

When you catch yourself thinking negative thoughts about your sleep, substitute more positive self-statements. Keep in mind a repertoire of realistic things to tell yourself when you feel discouraged. Here are some examples to consider:

- *"I've had a setback this week, but I'm doing a lot better than I used to. I just need to get back into good sleep habits."*

- *"I can't fall asleep, but I know it's because I stayed up late last night and slept in this morning. Next Sunday night will be better."*

- *"I can't get back to sleep, but at least I know to get up instead of lying here tossing and turning."*

- *"I've had two nights of insomnia, but if I keep getting up at my regular time, I'll be sleepy at bedtime before long."*

Don't just mouth or think statements like these. *Believe* them. A growing body of research has proved that insomnia is under your control. And keeping a positive attitude is one way to maintain your progress and keep from becoming discouraged.

WHEN IT DOESN'T COME EASILY

Your habits have been with you for years. Don't be surprised or discouraged if you occasionally slip back into old behaviors that interfere with sleep. Caffeine and alcohol use are everywhere in society. Stress, anxiety, and depression can grow without our awareness. Just one weekend of staying up late and sleeping in can throw our body rhythms out of sync with our sleep needs.

After you have completed this program, you may still have bouts of sleeplessness. But you will no longer panic when they occur. You will no longer feel victimized by insomnia or think that you are helpless to do anything about it.

You will know that you have the resources and the skills to improve your sleep. You will know how to prevent occasional sleep problems from becoming chronic and distressing. You will know that you're in control.

Appendices

Appendix 1
Relaxation Instructions

THIS APPENDIX INCLUDES INSTRUCTIONS FOR THREE TYPES OF relaxation introduced in Chapter 10 and further discussed in Chapter 15. There are many variations of relaxation instructions. These three work particularly well to help induce sleep at bedtime or after a nighttime awakening.

You can make your own audiotape of any or all of these exercises, then use the tape for "relaxation workouts." You may want to experiment a little before making a final tape, so the voice and phrasing feel right to you.

INSTRUCTIONS FOR TENSE-AND-RELEASE RELAXATION*

Note that a series of dots (...) does not mean that words are missing. Rather it indicates that you should pause for three to five seconds.

---

*These instructions were adapted from Joseph Wolpe, Ph.D., and Arnold Lazarus, Ph.D., *Behavior Therapy Techniques* (New York: Pergamon Press, 1966).

Settle back comfortably and gently close your eyes . . . Now, as you're relaxing, clench your right fist. Clench your fist tighter and tighter. Notice the tension as you do. Keep it clenched, and feel the tension in your right fist, hand, forearm . . . and now relax. Let the fingers of your right hand become loose, and observe the contrast in your feelings between the tension that was there a moment ago and the greater sense of relaxation now . . . Now once more clench your right fist really tight . . . Hold it, and notice the tension again . . . Now let go and relax. Let your fingers straighten out . . . Notice the difference once more . . . Okay, now we'll leave the right hand and move to the left hand.

Clench your left hand into a fist . . . very tense, very tight . . . Clench the fist tighter and notice the tension . . . and now relax. Again, notice the contrast . . . Repeat the tensing once more, clench the left fist, tight and tense . . . And now relax your hand. Continue relaxing like that for a while, both hands and fingers becoming more loose and relaxed.

Now we'll leave both hands comfortably relaxed and move to the right bicep. Bend your right arm at the elbow to tense your right bicep, the right upper arm . . . Tense them harder and notice the tightness . . . All right, now straighten out your arm. Let it relax and feel the difference again between tension and relaxation . . . Relaxation is the absence of tension. Okay, now once more tense your right bicep. Hold the tension and observe it carefully . . . And now straighten the arm and relax. Let your arm move to a comfortable position. Let the relaxation proceed on its own.

Now we'll move to the left bicep, the upper arm . . . Tense the upper arm by bending your left arm at the elbow, very tight, very tense . . . Feel the muscle tension in the bicep and the upper arm. All right, now release the tension. Let your arm return to a comfortable supported position, and notice the relaxation . . . Now once more, tense up the left upper arm, very tight . . . Notice the tension. This is how tenseness feels . . . And now relax the arm. Let the tension be replaced by relaxation, and let your arm move to a comfortably supported position.

So right now you can notice the increased sense of relaxation in the right hand . . . and the fingers of the right hand . . . and the right forearm . . . and also the right upper arm. Similarly, there is relaxation in the left hand . . . the fingers of the left hand . . . the left forearm . . . and the left upper arm. Very relaxed feelings in both hands and both arms . . . Now we'll leave both hands and arms comfortably supported and shift our attention to the area around the head.

We'll start at the forehead. Now wrinkle up your forehead. Wrinkle it tighter . . . as if you're frowning . . . tense, and tight . . . Now, relax the forehead and smooth it out. Picture the entire forehead becoming smoother as the relaxation increases . . . Now frown once more and wrinkle your brows and study the tension . . . very tight . . . Now let go of the tension and smooth out the forehead once more . . . Now we'll move to the eyes . . . Close your eyes tighter and tighter . . . feel the tension . . . Now relax your eyes; keeping your eyes closed, but comfortably relaxed . . . Notice the sense of relaxation . . . All right, once more, close your eyes really tight, and notice the tension . . . tight and tense . . . and now relax. Let the tension disappear and be replaced by a greater sense of relaxation, while your eyes are comfortably closed . . . much more relaxed.

Okay, we'll move now to the rest of the facial areas by having you clench your jaws . . . bite your teeth together. Study the tension throughout the jaws . . . All right now, relax your jaws . . . notice the relaxation all over your face . . . your forehead . . . your eyes, lips, and jaws . . . Now once more, bite your teeth, clench your jaws and notice the tension that creates . . . Okay, now relax the jaws and the entire facial area . . . Let the relaxation proceed on its own to cover the forehead, the eyes, the jaws, the entire facial area.

Now pay attention to your neck muscles. Press your head back as far as it can go and feel the tension in the neck . . . tense and tight . . . Now let your head return forward to a comfortable position, and notice the relaxation. Let the relaxation develop further . . . Once more, press your head back and notice the tension . . . All right, now relax the neck and let your head return to a comfortable position . . . Now we'll move to the shoulders . . . Shrug your shoulders, right up. Hold the tension . . . Drop your shoulders and feel the relaxation . . . Let the relaxation increase in the neck and shoulders . . . Shrug your shoulders again. Feel the tension in your shoulders and upper back . . . Now drop your shoulders once more and relax. Let the relaxation spread deep into the shoulders, right into your back muscles; relax your neck and shoulders . . . and your forehead and eyes . . . and the entire facial area. Now we'll move from the head and shoulders to your upper body.

Breathe easily and freely in and out. Notice how the relaxation has increased across your body . . . As you breathe comfortably, just feel that relaxation . . . Now inhale deeply and hold your breath. Study the tension . . . Now exhale. Let the walls of your chest grow loose and push the air out automatically. Continue relaxing, and breathe freely and easily. Feel the relaxation and enjoy it . . . Now breathe in deeply and hold it again . . . Just breathe out and appreciate the relief. Now breathe normally . . . Continue relaxing your chest, and let the relaxation spread to your shoulders, your neck, your facial area, and your arms. Merely let go . . . and enjoy the relaxation.

Now let's pay attention to your abdominal muscles, your stomach area. Tighten your stomach muscles, make your abdomen hard. Notice the tension . . . and relax. Let the muscles loosen and notice the contrast . . . Once more, press and tighten your stomach muscles. Hold the tension and pay attention to it . . . and relax. All right, we'll now move to your legs and feet.

To tense up your legs and feet, press your feet and toes downward, away from your body, so that your calf muscles become tense . . . just for a moment, so you don't get a cramp . . . All right, now relax. Allow the relaxation to proceed on its own . . . Now, once more, press your feet and toes downward, away from your face, so that your calf muscles become tense. Study how the tension feels . . . Okay, now relax your feet and legs.

Now you can become twice as relaxed as you are merely by taking in a really deep breath and slowly exhaling. Take in a long, deep breath, and let it out very slowly, using this method to become as relaxed as you would like to be. In the future we'll use this deep breath as a quick signal to achieve relaxation . . . Once more, take a deep breath and flow the relaxation across your body . . . relaxing your hands and arms . . . your facial area . . . the muscles of your neck and shoulders . . . your stomach . . . and both legs and both feet.

Just lie there and feel very calm. Notice the feelings of relaxation. In a moment, I'll count backward from three to one. When I get to one, open your eyes. You'll be calm and refreshed. All right . . . Three . . . feeling very calm . . . Two . . . very refreshed . . . One . . . feeling very calm.

INSTRUCTIONS FOR PASSIVE RELAXATION*

Note that each series of dots (. . .) indicates a pause of three to five seconds.

Settle back comfortably and gently close your eyes. Take a deep breath and hold it . . . Now let it out slowly. Take

---

*These instructions were adapted from those devised by James Ascough, Ph.D., Purdue University.

another deep breath and hold it . . . And let it out. Feelings of relaxation are beginning to spread to all parts of your body.

Now focus attention on your fingers and hands . . . Pay attention to the feelings in your hands and let go of the muscles. Relax the muscles in your hands . . . even more than you're doing now . . . Allow your fingers and hands to gradually become looser and heavier.

Let the relaxation begin to flow from the muscles of your fingers and hands . . . up through your forearms . . . Feel your forearms getting looser and heavier . . . Feel the relaxation that is now coming into your forearms . . . Your hands and forearms are getting looser and heavier . . . Let go of your muscles.

Take a slow deep breath and slowly exhale. Feel your body relaxing more and more . . . And return to breathing normally.

Now let go of the muscles in your upper arms and shoulders . . . a very heavy feeling coming into your arms and shoulders . . . getting more deeply relaxed . . . heavier . . . more relaxed . . . heavier . . . more relaxed . . . Just think of relaxing and you can feel the muscles getting looser . . . and heavier.

Now let the relaxation move up through your shoulders and into your neck . . . Your head is completely supported, so that your neck muscles can loosen . . . and relax . . . Let the neck muscles become loose . . . and relaxed . . . Let the muscles in your neck loosen . . . become limp . . . getting more and more relaxed.

Just like before, take a slow, deep breath and slowly exhale. Feel your body relaxing more and more . . . And return to breathing normally.

Now pay attention to your forehead . . . Smooth out your forehead . . . let the muscles become loose and limp . . . a heavy relaxed feeling spreading down from your forehead . . . and across your face . . . smooth and relaxed . . . Relax the muscles around your eyes . . . Let go of the muscles . . . Relax your cheeks . . . Your jaw muscles and the muscles around your mouth are also getting heavier and more relaxed . . . Feel them gradually becoming heavier and more relaxed.

The relaxation is spreading through your throat and neck . . . Just relax your chest . . . looser and more relaxed . . . Notice the muscles in your stomach . . . Feel those muscles getting looser . . . Think of letting go of those muscles . . . looser . . . and heavier . . . Now relax the muscles in your back . . . all the tightness leaving your back . . . Let the bed or chair completely support your back.

Take another slow deep breath and slowly exhale. Feel your body relaxing more and more . . . And return to breathing normally.

The muscles in your hips and thighs are getting looser and more relaxed . . . Feel how heavy your body has become . . . pressing down into the surface below. Just let yourself get heavier . . . looser . . . and more relaxed . . . Feel the wave of relaxation spreading through your body . . . heavier and more relaxed . . . Relaxation flowing down through your body . . . heavier and more relaxed . . . into your calves . . . Relax your calves . . . very deeply relaxed . . . your whole body still growing heavier . . . getting more relaxed.

Enjoy the feeling of deep relaxation that has spread to all parts of your body . . . Continue relaxing . . . deeper . . . and heavier . . . deeper . . . and heavier . . . deeper . . . and heavier.

Just lie there and feel very calm. Notice the feelings of relaxation. In a moment I'll count backward from three to one. When I get to one, open your eyes. You'll be calm and refreshed. All right . . . Three . . . feeling very calm . . . Two . . . refreshed . . . One . . . calm and refreshed.

INSTRUCTIONS FOR AUTOGENIC RELAXATION*

Note that each series of dots (...) indicates a pause of five to eight seconds. Each pause should last as long as the phrase preceding the pause, to allow yourself time to repeat the phrase in your mind.

During this type of relaxation there will be a statement followed by a pause. During that pause you think the same statement while attempting to experience what that statement describes. For example, the first statement is "My arms and legs are heavy and warm." Then there is a pause. It is during that pause that you think, "My arms and legs are heavy and warm," while you attempt to experience their *being* heavy and warm.

Most of those phrases will be repeated. Some will not. There will be some transitional phrases that will not be repeated. For example, "The relaxing warmth flows down to my right shoulder, and my right shoulder feels warm and heavy." The only thing you should repeat in your mind is "My right shoulder feels warm and heavy."

All right. Now take a deep breath and let it out slowly. Let yourself begin to relax all over.

My arms and legs are heavy and warm ... My arms and legs are heavy and warm ... My heartbeat is calm and regular ... My heartbeat is calm and regular ... My breathing is calm and regular ... My breathing is calm and regular ... My stomach is warm ... My stomach is warm ... My forehead is cool ... My forehead is cool ... My arms and legs are heavy and warm ... My heartbeat is calm and regular ... My breathing is calm and regular ... My stomach is warm ... My forehead is cool ... I am calm and re-

---

*These instructions were adapted by Fred Todd, Ph.D., of the Behavior Therapy Institute of Colorado, from the book by Neal Olshan and J. Wang, *Phobia-Free and Flying High* (Condor Publishing, 1978).

laxed . . . The top of my head feels warm and heavy . . .
The top of my head feels warm and heavy . . .

The relaxing warmth flows into my right shoulder, and
my right shoulder feels warm and heavy . . . My right
shoulder feels warm and heavy . . . All of the muscles in
my right shoulder are loose, limp, and slack . . . All of the
muscles in my right shoulder are loose, limp, and slack
. . . My breathing is getting deeper and deeper . . . The relaxing warmth flows down to my right hand, and my right
hand feels warm and heavy . . . My right hand feels warm
and heavy . . . All of the muscles in my right hand are
loose, limp, and slack . . . The relaxing warmth flows back
up into my right arm, and my right arm feels warm and
heavy . . . My right arm feels warm and heavy . . . All of the
muscles in my right arm are loose, limp, and slack . . . The
relaxing warmth spreads up through my right elbow into
my right shoulder, and my right elbow and shoulder feel
warm and heavy . . . My right elbow and shoulder feel
warm and heavy . . . All of the muscles in my right elbow and shoulder are loose, limp, and slack . . . The relaxing warmth flows slowly through my whole back; the
warmth is relaxing my back . . . My back feels warm and
heavy . . . My back feels warm and heavy . . . All of the
muscles in my back are loose, limp, and slack . . . The relaxing warmth moves up my back into my neck, and my
neck feels warm and heavy . . . My neck feels warm and
heavy . . . All of the muscles in my neck are loose, limp,
and slack . . . All of the muscles in my neck are loose, limp,
and slack . . . The relaxing warmth flows into my left
shoulder, and my left shoulder feels warm and heavy . . .
My left shoulder feels warm and heavy . . . All of the muscles in my left shoulder are loose, limp, and slack . . . All
of the muscles in my left shoulder are loose, limp, and
slack . . . My breathing is getting deeper and deeper . . .
The relaxing warmth flows down into my left hand, and
my left hand feels warm and heavy . . . All of the muscles
in my left hand are loose, limp, and slack . . . All of the

muscles in my left hand are loose, limp, and slack . . . The relaxing warmth flows back up to my left arm, and my left arm feels warm and heavy . . . My left arm feels warm and heavy . . . All of the muscles in my left arm are loose, limp, and slack . . . All of the muscles in my left arm are loose, limp, and slack . . . The relaxing warmth gradually flows up my left elbow through my left shoulder, and my left shoulder and elbow feel warm and heavy . . . My left shoulder and elbow feel warm and heavy . . . All of the muscles in my left elbow and shoulder are loose, limp, and slack . . . All of the muscles in my left elbow and shoulder are loose, limp, and slack . . .

The relaxing warmth flows to my heart, and my heart feels warm and easy . . . My heart feels warm and easy . . . My heartbeat is calm and regular . . . My heartbeat is calm and regular . . . The relaxing warmth flows down into my stomach, and my stomach feels warm . . . My stomach feels warm . . . My breathing is deeper and deeper . . . My breathing is calm and regular . . .

The relaxing warmth flows down into my right thigh, and my right thigh feels warm and heavy . . . My right thigh feels warm and heavy . . . All of the muscles in my right thigh are loose, limp, and slack . . . All of the muscles in my right thigh are loose, limp, and slack . . . The relaxing warmth flows down into my right foot, and my right foot feels warm and heavy . . . My right foot feels warm and heavy . . . All of the muscles in my right foot are loose, limp, and slack . . . All of the muscles in my right foot are loose, limp, and slack . . . The relaxing warmth flows slowly up through my right calf to my right knee to my right thigh, and my right leg feels warm and heavy . . . My right leg feels warm and heavy . . . All of the muscles in my right leg are loose, limp, and slack . . . All of the muscles in my right leg are loose, limp, and slack . . . My breathing is deeper and deeper . . . My breathing is deeper and deeper . . .

The relaxing warmth flows down into my left thigh, and

my left thigh feels warm and heavy . . . My left thigh feels warm and heavy . . . All of the muscles in my left thigh are loose, limp, and slack . . . All of the muscles in my left thigh are loose, limp, and slack . . . The relaxing warmth flows down into my left foot, and my left foot feels warm and heavy . . . My left foot feels warm and heavy . . . All of the muscles in my left foot are loose, limp, and slack . . . All of the muscles in my left foot are loose, limp, and slack . . . The relaxing warmth flows slowly up my left calf to my left knee and my left thigh, and my left leg feels warm and heavy . . . My left leg feels warm and heavy . . . All of the muscles in my left leg are loose, limp, and slack . . . All of the muscles in my left leg are loose, limp, and slack . . .

My breathing is deeper and deeper . . . My breathing is deeper and deeper . . . The relaxing warmth moves up through my stomach into my heart, and my heart feels warm . . . My heart feels warm . . . I am calm and relaxed . . . I am calm and relaxed . . .

Now just remain in that position, enjoying the feelings of relaxation, the feelings of heaviness and warmth, of calmness and relaxation . . . In a moment I'll count backward from three to one. When I get to one, open your eyes. You'll be calm and refreshed. All right . . . Three . . . feeling very calm . . . Two . . . feeling refreshed . . . One . . . calm and refreshed.

Appendix 2
Mental Imagery: A Sample Scene

HERE IS A DETAILED SCENE THAT YOU CAN USE TO CREATE calming and relaxing images in your mind. You can use these images as a daytime stress-management technique, as in Chapter 10, or to help induce sleep at bedtime, as in Chapter 15.

This scene may be used as a model for constructing your own relaxing mental images. Mental imagery scenes can be whatever you want them to be. They can be realistic, modeled on a memory from a vacation or a place from your childhood. They can be fanciful; for example, you can imagine floating on a cloud. Or they can combine realistic and imaginative elements — for example, floating slowly on an inner tube down a warm stream, with birds singing and crickets chirping.

If you decide to create your own relaxing mental images, it is a good idea to arrange a special private entryway into the scene, such as a path or staircase. Fill the scene with details using all the senses, not only sight but sound, scent, taste, and touch. Create a foreground and a background. Make your special place peaceful, safe, and comfortable.

A BEACH SCENE

Note that each series of dots (. . .) indicates a pause of two to five seconds.

Imagine yourself walking slowly down a long white-washed wooden stairway . . . The stairway ends at an open, expansive beach that stretches as far as you can see . . . The sky is a deep blue, with billowy white clouds blocking the sun's heat . . . The beach is deserted except for a few children playing off in the distance . . .

As you step off the stairway, feel the clean white sand . . . It is firm, yet it gives a little as your feet sink in . . . The sand moves between your toes . . . You move your feet and wiggle your toes to savor the softness of the sand . . .

Now you turn toward the ocean . . . The clean salt breeze blows gently against your face . . . tickles your nose . . . It feels cool and refreshing . . . Yet the sun above warms you and makes you feel very comfortable . . . You walk slowly along the sand . . .

Far away you hear roaring surf . . . It soothes away any tension you feel . . . Just in front of you, waves gently lap against the shore . . . They ebb and flow rhythmically . . . Farther out, sunlight plays along the whitecaps . . . You feel calm as you notice the deep blue shade of the ocean itself . . . You look out over the surface of the ocean . . . all the way to the horizon . . .

In the distance a sailboat skims easily along the surface of the water . . . For a moment you think you can hear the flapping of its sails in the breeze . . . But then you hear the sound of birds . . . You look up and see two sea gulls soaring down the beach . . . They turn and fly out to sea . . . The gulls are graceful as they soar . . . You imagine what it would feel like to fly . . .

As you walk along slowly, the sea breeze continues to

waft slowly over your cheeks and neck . . . It ruffles your hair . . . The sun warms your shoulders, your hair, your hands . . . The salt air feels moist and clean as you slowly breathe in . . . and out . . . You feel more and more content . . .

Now you come to a stretch of low sand dunes . . . Tufts of grass are swaying in the breeze . . . They brush against your legs . . . You walk among the dunes . . . On an impulse you lie down in the sand . . . Its warmth cradles your body as you settle in . . . You close your eyes . . . becoming more and more relaxed . . . nestling into the sand . . . The sun above and the sand below fill your body with warmth . . . You feel heavier and warmer . . . warmer and heavier . . .

Soft breezes play all around you . . . The gentle rhythm of the surf carries you deeper into relaxation . . . You feel warm . . . cozy . . . comfortable . . . at peace.

Appendix 3
Night Work

MORE THAN SEVEN MILLION AMERICANS WORK THE NIGHT shift or rotate among day, evening, and night shifts. These people suffer frequently from sleep problems. One survey showed that 60 percent of night workers complain of disturbed sleep. Reports of poor sleep have been validated by scientific studies showing that shift workers do have shortened and disrupted sleep, as well as increased sleepiness when not in bed. Sleep problems commonly experienced by night workers include difficulty falling asleep, poor-quality sleep, chronic fatigue, excessive use of caffeine and tobacco to keep alert, and sleepiness at work.

You may recall from Chapter 11 that our bodies' circadian rhythms are tied intricately to the rising and setting of the sun. The invention of the light bulb in 1879 made night work possible. As a consequence, many people were forced to schedule their lives around their job demands rather than nature's cycle of light and darkness.

If a person with difficulty adjusting to night work consults a sleep specialist, the first recommendation will be the obvious one: Get a day job. But this isn't always possible. Let's look at some guidelines for minimizing night work's negative effects on sleep.

NIGHT SHIFT

The night shift goes from about 11:00 P.M. to 7:00 A.M. The best way to adjust your body's circadian rhythms to night work is to maintain the same sleep-wake schedule seven days a week. People who follow this strategy typically adapt well to night work. They feel alert at night and sleep soundly during the day.

However, few night workers follow this strategy, because they prefer to socialize on a conventional schedule on their days off. If you are a night worker, there are several steps you can take to improve your sleep, whether or not you switch to conventional hours on your days off work:

- *Schedule your sleep time, and defend it from interruptions. Don't let visitors or phone calls wake you.*

- *Make your bedroom as dark and soundproof as you can. Review the ideas in Chapter 13 about setting up your sleep environment.*

- *Be careful about alcohol, tobacco, and caffeine, which can disrupt sleep (see Chapter 8).*

- *Wear dark, wraparound sunglasses when you leave work and drive home, to prevent morning sunlight from entering your retinas and alerting your brain's internal clock that it is time to be awake. Use blinds or draperies to make sure that no daylight penetrates your bedroom when you lie down to sleep.*

  Light therapy (Chapter 11) can adjust your body clock to the sleep-wake schedule you need to follow. A 1990 study published in the New England Journal of Medicine *by the research group at Harvard Medical School's Center for Circadian and Sleep Disorders Medicine exposed night workers for four nights to bright light, using light boxes ranging from 7,000 to 12,000 lux. They succeeded in changing the body temperature's low point (when the body is sleepiest) from 3:30 A.M. to 3:00 P.M. Subjects slept an average of two hours a day longer when receiving light therapy at night.*

- *Consider napping. Because most night workers sleep fewer hours than other people, they tend to be chronically sleep-deprived. A nap can help compensate for lost sleep.*

ROTATING SHIFTS

People who work day, evening, and night shifts experience "blue-collar jet lag," so named because rotating through work shifts is like flying across the Earth's time zones. One survey of rotating shift workers showed that more than half admitted to falling asleep at work.

You will function best if your shifts rotate in a forward direction, from day shift to evening to night shift. The body's internal clock can adjust more easily to a shift rotation in this direction because days are pushed forward and extended, corresponding to the body's preference for a twenty-five-hour day. Most industries have traditionally rotated workers through shifts in the opposite direction: from day to night to evening. Many employers have reversed their schedules so that they now rotate forward. Some, however, have not.

If you work a shift that rotates forward, you can give your internal clock a head start in adjusting to the next shift. A few days before your shift changes, begin staying up a little later and sleeping in later. This phase delay will help your body prepare for the new shift so you can ease into it more smoothly.

Appendix 4
Jet Lag

JET LAG IS THE TEMPORARY MALADJUSTMENT YOU EXPERI-
ence when a rapid change of time zones causes your internal biological rhythms to become out of phase with
the new local time. Symptoms of jet lag can include daytime fatigue and sleepiness, gastrointestinal problems, and
insomnia.

The severity of jet lag depends on how many time zones
you cross and how quickly you cross them. Difficulty adjusting is much less pronounced when you cross just one
or two time zones. When you travel slowly by car or ship,
jet lag will be mild or nonexistent. And north-south travel
does not cause jet lag, because time zones do not vary from
north to south.

Most people adjust more easily to westbound travel, because it extends the day's length. As you learned in Chapter 11, a longer day corresponds to the body's preference
for a twenty-five-hour day. Research has compared the effects of westbound and eastbound travel across six time

zones between America and Europe. Travelers have been found to take just three days to adjust to westbound flights but nine days to adjust to eastbound flights.

Remember that the body's circadian rhythms tend to shorten in old age, from twenty-five hours to twenty-four hours or less. Because of this normal developmental change, older adults find it easier to adjust to eastward air travel and harder to adjust to westward air travel, compared with young or middle-aged adults.

Two alternative strategies can help you minimize the effects of jet lag.

WHEN TO STAY ON HOME TIME

Sleeping on your home time instead of adjusting to a new time zone is the best way to minimize jet lag. Airline pilots often follow this strategy: They eat and sleep by watches set on their home times. Usually this is feasible only for brief trips of a few days or less.

In this approach, you need to schedule events at times when you would be awake and alert at home. For example, an American in Europe should try to schedule meetings in the late afternoon, corresponding to morning hours in the United States.

The same principle can be applied to coast-to-coast travel. A New Yorker traveling to California should try to schedule events before about 2:00 P.M. Pacific time. Conversely, a Californian traveling to the East Coast should schedule events in the afternoon on Eastern Time.

WHEN TO ADJUST TO THE NEW TIME ZONE

For trips longer than a few days it may be impractical to stay on home time. In these instances, the following suggestions can help you adjust quickly and efficiently to a new time zone.

- Begin adjusting before you leave home. *You can take steps before you leave home to minimize jet lag, by gradually adjusting your sleep hours to the time zone of your destination. For example, if you plan to travel from New York to California, go to bed later on the nights before the trip, and sleep in later. To prepare yourself for eastbound travel, set your alarm to wake up earlier for a few mornings before you leave. This earlier waking hour will make it easier to go to sleep earlier on the nights before your trip.*

- Drink fluids on the plane, but avoid alcohol and caffeine. *Special diets have been proposed as ways to prevent or reduce jet lag. There is no evidence that any of these diets makes a real difference. However, it is important to drink plenty of fluids to prevent dehydration in the low humidity of a pressurized airplane cabin, because dehydration worsens the effects of jet lag. Avoiding alcohol and caffeine is helpful; these drugs aggravate dehydration and add stress to your body that makes it harder for your internal rhythms to adjust to time changes.*

- Arrive early. *If you are traveling across time zones for an important event, arriving several days early will help you get over the worst effects of jet lag before the event.*

- Switch immediately to the new time zone. *When you reach your destination, don't go to bed just because you feel sleepy. Instead, wait until it is bedtime in your new time zone. Conversely, get up in the morning at your local wake-up time, even if your body doesn't feel ready.*

  Go outside and get as much sunshine as you can, especially in the early morning. As noted in Chapter 11, sunlight is a powerful stimulus for adjusting the body's circadian rhythms.

Appendix 5
Help Your Child Sleep Through the Night

IF YOU READ BOOKS ON CHILD CARE OR ASK FRIENDS, RELA-
tives, or professionals about your child's sleep problem, be
prepared to contend with conflicting advice. In most instances, there is no "right" answer that applies to all children. When you hear different recommendations, don't
worry about which is the "correct" one. No solution is
perfect, and different approaches sometimes work best
with different children. You have to choose what you think
will work for *your* child. With your child, you are the
expert.

HOW TO PREVENT CHILDREN'S SLEEP PROBLEMS

Some children fall asleep easily and sleep soundly through
the night. Others regularly have difficulty falling asleep,
staying asleep, or both. Part of this difference appears to
reflect inherited genetic abilities. However, any infant or
child can learn positive sleep habits to improve sleep.

GUIDELINES FOR INFANTS

1. Help your baby learn that the night is for sleeping. A newborn typically sleeps in six to eight intervals off and on around the clock. Over the first three months, infants begin to develop a day-night wake-sleep rhythm. By about six months, 80 percent babies sleep well through the night. However, about 10 percent do not establish a consistent day-night wake-sleep pattern until they are more than a year old.

   You can establish a regular rhythm that will help your baby fall asleep and stay asleep at night. Regularly show your baby the difference between day and night by exposure to light and darkness cycles. Provide plenty of sunshine, music, and stimulation during the day. Don't let a nap go on for more than about three consecutive hours; after that, wake your baby gently.

   It is a good idea to begin a pleasant and predictable bedtime routine when your baby is only a few months old. By age one, a familiar bedtime routine is very important. As with adults, a bedtime routine can take on a ritual quality that is comforting and sleep-inducing. A bedtime routine for an infant can be as simple as reading a book such as *Goodnight Moon*, saying good night, turning out the light, laying baby in the crib, and singing a lullaby. Older children often respond well to a more involved bedtime routine, as noted below.

   Keep the baby's room dark and quiet at night. At feedings and changings, don't talk except to tell your baby to go back to sleep afterward. Do everything you can to help your infant think of the night as a special time for sleeping.

2. Hold your baby in a front carrier during the day. Research has shown that young infants do only half their usual bedtime fussing and crying when they get to ride in a front carrier for at least three hours during the day or evening.

3. Lengthen the time between daytime feedings, and reduce nighttime feedings. When older infants are fed too frequently, their stomachs become conditioned to expect frequent feedings. When your infant is three to six months old, try lengthening the interval between daytime feedings to four hours or more.

   Make middle-of-the-night feedings as brief as you can. By age two months, most children are down to one nighttime feeding around 2:00 A.M. At that age, consider reducing your baby's formula by one or two ounces or spending a shorter time nursing than you would during the day. See if holding the baby without feeding provides comfort.

   Try to eliminate all nighttime feeding by four or five months. At this age, most infants need to be fed only four times a day (five times for nursing babies), so hunger is less likely to wake them at night.

4. Teach your child to fall asleep alone and without your help. Until infants are three to six months old, they need to be comforted whenever they cry during the day or night. But when they settle down, they should be put in the crib *before* falling asleep. This will help your child learn the skill of falling asleep in the crib, alone and without your help. Your child can then use this skill to return to sleep after waking during the night. Remember, awakenings during the night are frequent for children as well as adults. What is crucial is for children to learn to fall back asleep on their own.

   Let's say your daughter is seven months old. When you leave her in bed, be sure she is drowsy but still awake. Her last waking memory should be of lying alone in the crib or bed. In that way, she will not come to associate falling asleep with you or with being fed. Instead she will associate falling asleep with lying alone in her crib. This guideline helps develop good sleep habits important for infants, toddlers, and pre-schoolers.

It is all right to rub or nurse her to sleep if she normally sleeps well through the night. But if she has trouble sleeping, do not let her fall asleep while she is being fed or rubbed or held. If you do, she will learn to associate those external comforts with falling asleep. Then, to fall asleep initially or to return to sleep from a nighttime awakening, she will need to be touched or fed. Instead, leave her alone before she falls asleep.

If she cries at bedtime and after nighttime awakenings, allow her to cry alone for about five minutes. Then go in to check her, but stay for no more than a minute. Staying longer may reinforce the crying and encourage more. But a brief visit will reassure her that she has not been abandoned, and it will reassure you that she is all right.

You may want to wipe her nose and check that she is not wet, but don't pick her up or otherwise reinforce the crying. Gently call her by name and tell her to go to sleep. Then leave. If the crying continues, wait about fifteen minutes, because often an infant will return to sleep after ten to fifteen minutes of crying. Then go in again. Wipe her face and tell her to go to sleep; then leave again while she is still awake. Return to check on her every fifteen minutes, as many times as necessary.

The regimen described above was developed by pediatrician Barton Schmitt of the University of Colorado School of Medicine and Children's Hospital in Denver. Different authorities use different regimens and lengths of time before checking. Pediatrician Richard

Ferber uses a progressive schedule in which the intervals between checks increase in length with each passing night. This is Ferber's recommended schedule for checking on a crying child at night:

Day 1: Wait five minutes before the first check. Then wait ten minutes before the second check and fifteen minutes before each subsequent check.

Day 2: Wait ten minutes before the first check. Then wait fifteen minutes before the second check and twenty minutes before each subsequent check.

Day 3: Wait fifteen minutes before the first check. Then wait twenty minutes before the second check and twenty-five minutes before each subsequent check.

In Ferber's program, you continue the above progression by adding five minutes to each interval on successive nights.

Whichever schedule is used, children typically cry an hour or two the first night and thirty to sixty minutes the second night. Because parents will lose sleep on the first nights of this approach, it's best to begin treatment on the weekend. The child will cry less on each successive night. By the seventh night most children learn to fall asleep by themselves.

Other authorities recommend different approaches. Pediatricians T. Berry Brazelton and Marianne Neifert suggest that after going to a child several times, a parent just call out reassuringly instead of entering the bedroom. Because there is no single best way, you should devise a plan that you are comfortable with and that you think will work for your child.

Regardless of the particular approach you use, by about age six months it is a good idea to encourage your baby to choose a favorite soft toy — such as a stuffed animal — to sleep with. He or she will learn to associate lying alone next to this companion with falling asleep. Then, when the baby awakens during the night, the stuffed toy will serve as a comforting cue to help induce sleep.

Some parents choose to postpone teaching their children to fall asleep by themselves until they are older and more independent. Instead, they sleep together with their young children in a family bed. This practice will be examined later in the chapter.

GUIDELINES FOR PRESCHOOL AND SCHOOL-AGE CHILDREN

1. Limit naps. Children show large individual differences in how often and for how long they nap, as well as when they give up napping. Children outgrow their morning naps between ages one and one half and two and their afternoon naps between three and six.

   Try to get your child down for a nap by early afternoon, and limit the nap to two hours. Otherwise your child will be too alert to fall asleep at bedtime.

2. Make sure that your child gets plenty of exercise. There are two sleep-related reasons to encourage active outside play. First, good all-around exercise and fitness help establish sound sleep. Second, for a child with trouble falling asleep or sleeping through the night, it is particularly good to exercise hard about four to six hours before bedtime, just as we saw with adults in Chapter 14.

3. Be careful about caffeine. Cola and other caffeinated drinks can easily cause insomnia in children. When a child drinks a can of cola or other caffeinated soda pop, the caffeine intake is roughly equivalent to four cups of coffee for an adult. It is best to avoid caffeine entirely, but if you allow your child to have chocolate or caffeinated drinks, limit it to earlier than six hours before bedtime.

4. Help your child wind down during the evening. With children as with adults, it is important to use the evening as a time of quiet transition between wakefulness and sleep. Encourage your child to finish homework and other stimulating activities by a few hours before bedtime. During the evening, relaxing activities such as reading and quiet play are best.

5. Set up a bedtime routine that encourages drowsiness and sleep. A familiar bedtime routine gives children a sense of security and helps them to associate bedtime with sleepiness. A typical bedtime routine for a child can include any of these or similar activities:

- *Brushing teeth*
- *Using the toilet*
- *Taking a bath*
- *Putting on pajamas*
- *Closing the bedroom shades or curtains*
- *Saying prayers*
- *Listening to a bedtime story*
- *Saying good night to stuffed toys*
- *Lying down and being covered*
- *Turning off the lights*
- *Good-night hug and kiss*
- *Good-night song*

Design a routine that works for you and your child. Follow the different steps in the same order each night. A good bedtime routine usually takes about thirty minutes.

Keep one point in mind when you set up a bedtime routine for your child. Children can be frightened by the prayer with the words "If I should die before I wake," so it's best to choose another.

Around age nine or ten many children begin to want privacy before they go to bed. Respect this normal developmental change, and allow your child to go through much of the routine alone.

6. Keep bedtime a positive experience. If the bedtime routine is pleasant, your child will look forward to bedtime rather than resent it.

If your child isn't sleepy at bedtime, allow a low light and a book to read. Switch on a night-light or keep the bedroom door open, if this helps your child feel safer and more relaxed.

Don't put children to bed as a punishment. Disciplining children by sending them to bed will cause them to feel negatively about bed and sleep. Instead, confine them to their rooms for a period of time, or choose a different consequence.

7. Consider a later bedtime for your child. As parents, we expect our children to be unique, and we enjoy their distinctive qualities. Yet many parents think that all children at a given age have the same sleep needs. Don't assume that your child needs the average sleep requirement for his or her age. Just as with adults, there is a wide range in sleep requirements among children of the same age.

The table below shows how long children typically sleep at different ages. However, it does not show how long *your* child needs to sleep. It includes the range in which two out of three children at different ages sleep each day, including naps.

Average Daily Sleep of Children (in Hours)

AGE	TOTAL SLEEP TIME	RANGE*
1 week	16.3	14–18
3 months	15.0	13–17
6 months	13.7	11.7–15.5
1 year	13.2	11.4–15
2 years	12.5	11–13.3
4 years	11.3	10.5–12
6 years	11.0	10–11.5
10 years	10.0	9–11
15 years	9.0	7–11

*Two-thirds of children sleep this amount. One in six sleeps less, and one in six sleeps more.

Adapted from *A Good Night's Sleep* by Jerrold Maxmen (New York: W. W. Norton & Co., 1981). Copyright © 1981. Adapted by permission of W. W. Norton & Co.

Don't worry about whether your child is getting enough sleep. Psychologist Wilse Webb spent a lifetime researching human sleep needs and the effects of sleep deprivation. When parents asked him how much sleep their child needed, he would reply, "I can't answer you, but your child can." That is, when a child needs sleep, he or she will sleep. A child who is alert during the day is getting enough sleep at night.

Not all authorities agree on this issue. Some say that you should require your child to stay in bed the average sleep requirement for the child's age. Decide what seems best for your child. With your child, *you* are the real expert.

8. Help your child establish a regular sleep-wake schedule. Remember, it is helpful for adults to go to bed at the same time each night and even more important for them to get up at the same time each day. Like

adults, children sleep best when they follow these two principles.

Many older children and adolescents sleep in late whenever they can. This throws their internal clock off its rhythm and often leads to Sunday-night insomnia.

Getting your child up at the same time each morning leads to sleepiness at a regular time each night. Like an adult, a child will establish a regular internal rhythm and maintain a regular sleep-wake schedule if he or she gets up around the same time each morning.

For most children it is best to go to bed at the same time each night. However, some parents find that it is better to let their children stay up until they are sleepy. Do what seems right for you.

WHAT ABOUT THE FAMILY BED?

In the past, nearly all parents slept with their young children in one bed, as is still the custom in most parts of the world today. Around the fifteenth century, the idea of the private bedroom was invented in Europe, and some parents began to keep their children out of their beds and require them to sleep alone.

In Western industrialized nations, particularly the United States, this trend accelerated during the eighteenth and nineteenth centuries. Religious forces and advocates of discipline and self-reliance began a movement to keep children out of their parents' beds. Since then, many American parents have required their children to sleep alone. However, a 1984 survey published in the journal *Pediatrics* reported that 35 percent of white families and 70 percent of black families allow children under four years old to sleep in their parents' beds.

Many parents believe that sleeping with their young children promotes security and family closeness while causing no negative effects. In 1976, a counselor for the La Leche League named Tine Thevenin wrote *The Family Bed* (copyright © 1976 by Tine Thevenin, Minneapolis, MN), an important book that first examined this approach systematically. Since that time, some respected authorities — such as pediatrician T. Berry Brazelton — have reversed their initial criticism of this practice and now conclude that it is all right for a family to sleep together.

Chapter 15 points out that no one sleeps well in a crowded bed, because one person's movements can disturb the sleep of another. Some families who try sleeping together in one bed feel crowded and experience disturbed sleep. However, others have no problem. Using a king-size bed will increase the likelihood that a family will sleep well together.

Those who disapprove of children sleeping with their parents usually speculate about problems with lack of independence or sexual confusion that children may develop. Pediatrician Richard Ferber writes: "Sleeping alone is an important part of [your child's] learning to separate from you without anxiety and to see himself as an independent individual." In response, pediatrician William Sears states in the book *Nighttime Parenting* (New York: Plume, 1985):

How often have you heard, "But the baby will get to enjoy it; he'll become so dependent that he'll never want to leave your bed"? Yes, of course the baby will enjoy it. Is there anything in the parent-child contract that says your baby shouldn't enjoy where he sleeps? Yes, he will temporarily seem dependent and not want to leave your bed. This is a natural consequence of the feeling of rightness. When you're close to someone you love and you feel right, why give that up?

You are not encouraging dependency when you sleep with your baby. . . . In my experience children who are given open access to the family bed in infancy become more secure and independent in the long run. They reach the stage of independence when they are ready.

Another potential problem raised by Ferber is this: "If your child always sleeps with you, you may have great difficulty leaving him with a sitter." However, parents who use a family bed typically find that this is not a problem. Their children separate readily from them to stay with a baby-sitter or at a day-care center.

When children mature to the developmental level at which they want more privacy, peer interaction, and independence from their parents, they typically choose to begin sleeping alone in their own beds. Because they are older and better able to control their behavior, they can learn to fall asleep readily by themselves — especially if you help them develop positive sleep habits with the eight guidelines for older children outlined in the previous section.

In her book *Dr. Mom* (New York: Signet, 1987), pediatrician Marianne Neifert offers her professional opinion: "The family bed is a personal decision, not anyone else's concern, and is a healthy and restful way to sleep while parenting young children."

There is no evidence that a parent or parents sharing a bed with young children is harmful in any way. With this family issue, do what makes you comfortable and what feels right for you and your child.

OTHER CHILDHOOD SLEEP PROBLEMS AND WHAT TO DO ABOUT THEM

Like adults, children can suffer from poor sleep as the result of medical problems. Among young children, common physical causes of sleeplessness include wet or soiled bedclothes, teething, colic and other gastrointestinal disorders, tonsil and adenoid enlargement, and ear infections. Be sure to discuss any concerns about your child's sleep with the doctor, to consider possible medical causes.

NIGHTMARES

Help your child understand that dreams are make-believe, like a TV show. When your child awakens after a nightmare, offer reassurance by telling the child that he or she is all right and just had a bad dream. It can be helpful to share the fact that you have nightmares sometimes, too. Asking the question "How scared are you?" helps children know that you want to understand and are not going to dismiss their fears.

Sometimes children with nightmares will calm down if you encourage them to replace bad thoughts with good ones. For example, have them name all the things that make them happy, or figure out how to end the dream in a safe or humorous way.

NIGHT TERRORS

As noted in Chapter 2, night terrors occur during incomplete awakening from the deepest level of sleep. These half-awake panic reactions often happen within the first hour after falling asleep, and almost always within the first four hours of sleep. Two or three children out of a hundred — more boys than girls — have night terrors. They are most common in children three to five years old, and they usually disappear as the child grows older.

A child experiencing a night terror is still really sleeping and cannot readily understand or talk to you. Don't intervene in a night terror. Trying to soothe or wake a child may increase agitation and prolong the episode. In most cases the child falls back asleep within fifteen minutes and the next day has no memory of what happened.

Getting overtired can trigger a night terror, because a very tired child will sleep more deeply. Chapter 2 shows that you can prevent sleep terrors in a child prone to them by arranging for him or her to sleep longer. This will reduce deep sleep, during which night terrors occur.

Another approach is to notice for several nights how many minutes typically pass from the child's falling asleep to the onset of the sleep terror. Then wake the child fifteen minutes before a night terror may be due. Repeat this for seven consecutive nights.

SLEEPWALKING

Sleepwalking is relatively common in children. About 15 percent of children sleepwalk at least once, compared with 3 or 4 percent of adults. As with night terrors, sleepwalking usually is outgrown by late adolescence. Boys are more likely than girls to sleepwalk.

As noted in Chapter 2, you should try to protect a sleepwalker from injury by taking preventive measures, such as locking outside doors and blocking stairways.

NARCOLEPSY

As you learned from Chapter 2, narcolepsy is a disorder that causes irresistible daytime sleepiness. Narcolepsy can start as early as age ten. If your child shows any signs of this disorder, discuss your concerns with the doctor. If you have further concerns, you can contact the professional staff of a sleep disorders center (see Appendix 6).

SLEEP APNEA

Although this breathing disorder occurs mostly in older adults, children can suffer from apnea as well. Often this problem is related to enlarged tonsils or adenoids. If your child snores loudly or has difficulty breathing during sleep, discuss the problem and what to do about it with the doctor.

BED-WETTING

Bed-wetting, or *enuresis*, is a common childhood problem. About 15 percent of five-year-olds, 5 percent of ten-year-olds, and 1 to 2 percent of adolescents still wet their beds. As with many childhood behavior problems, boys are more likely than girls to wet the bed.

It is a myth that bed-wetting is caused by emotional problems. According to the National Institute of Mental Health fewer than 1 percent of bed-wetting cases have an emotional cause. Most cases of bed-wetting are caused by a congenitally small bladder, a bladder infection, or another physical problem.

Heredity contributes greatly to bed-wetting. A child with one parent who wet the bed during childhood has a 45 percent chance of developing enuresis. If both parents wet their beds during childhood, the probability increases to 75 percent.

In some cases, bed-wetting can be prevented by reducing excessive fluid intake during the evening and waking the child during the night. If you get your child up to urinate, be sure that he or she is fully awake, to avoid strengthening the association between sleep and urination.

There are two major methods of treating bed-wetting behaviorally. You can help children develop control of their bladder muscles by encouraging them to drink a lot of fluids during the day and rewarding them for holding urine for progressively longer periods. Stream-interruption exercises, in which a child voluntarily starts and stops urine flow, can also help develop bladder control.

The second behavioral approach is to condition your child — that is, to change the behavior that serves as a stimulus for the urination response. Commercially available devices sound an alarm when the child urinates and wets a sensor attached to the underwear. In this way, the child learns, or is conditioned, to associate bladder feelings just before urination with the need to awaken. A review of forty different studies with more than one thousand children showed a 75 percent success rate with this method.

CHILDHOOD-ONSET INSOMNIA

We saw in Chapter 2 that a small number of children are subject to severe insomnia. This sleep problem can be part of a neurological syndrome that often — but not always — involves hyperactivity and learning disabilities as well.

If you suspect your child has childhood-onset insomnia, it is especially important to follow all the methods that help other children prevent sleep problems. In addition, consider talking to your child's doctor about the possibility of an evaluation at a sleep disorders center (see Appendix 6).

IF YOU NEED FURTHER HELP

Every book on child care includes information and suggestions regarding sleep and sleep problems. The sleep section in pediatrician Barton Schmitt's *Your Child's Health* (New York: Bantam, 1991) is particularly enlightening. A comprehensive source of information is the book *Solve Your Child's Sleep Problems* (New York: Fireside [Simon & Schuster], 1985) by pediatrician Richard Ferber.

If your child has a sleep problem you can't solve on your own, ask the doctor for advice. Your child's doctor can help you design an individual plan to help your child sleep better. Alternatively, you may want to consult a mental health professional who has expertise in behavioral methods of solving children's sleep problems.

Appendix 6
Sleep Disorders Centers

THERE ARE TWO SITUATIONS IN WHICH YOU MIGHT NEED professional help to solve your sleep problem. First, because insomnia and poor sleep may have medical causes, ask your doctor about any possible physical reasons for your sleep problem.

Second, if stress, anxiety, or depression may be interfering with your sleep, and if you have not benefited from self-help methods to reduce problems in one of those areas, you may want to consult a mental-health professional. Use the methods discussed at the end of Chapter 9 for selecting a counselor or therapist.

In addition, there are several situations in which an evaluation at a sleep disorders center may be necessary.

WHEN TO GO TO A SLEEP DISORDERS CENTER

There are three problems for which you should consider being evaluated at a sleep disorders center. The first is if

you or your bed partner notices that you may have con-
stricted breathing or excessive leg movements during
sleep. Second, excessive daytime sleepiness can be caused
by several medical factors that are detectable only by an
evaluation at a sleep disorders center. Third, you should
consider this kind of evaluation if you suffer from severe
and relentless insomnia that impairs your daytime functioning and has not improved despite genuine efforts to
change possible causes such as mental health problems,
medical conditions, or the kinds of sleep-related habits reviewed in Part IV.

HOW TO FIND A SLEEP DISORDERS CENTER

You can contact the American Sleep Disorders Association to obtain a list of accredited centers:

American Sleep Disorders Association
1610 Fourteenth Street N.W., Suite 300
Rochester, MN 55901
Telephone: 507-287-6006

Accreditation ensures that a center meets the rigorous professional standards of this association.

If there is no accredited center nearby, try calling large
hospitals and medical schools in your area. Many medical
facilities have sleep disorders centers that may not be fully
accredited but can nonetheless provide a valid and professional evaluation of sleep problems.

If you want to be evaluated at a sleep disorders center,
ask your physician to make a referral. Alternatively, you
can contact a sleep disorders center directly and discuss
the referral process with one of its staff members. In 1993
the charge for an evaluation at a sleep disorders center,
including a night sleeping in the lab, averages about fifteen
hundred dollars; costs vary depending on the center and
on the different tests ordered. Medical insurance policies

typically cover the cost of a sleep evaluation if medical specialists certify that one is required.

At the sleep disorders center, you will be asked to complete a questionnaire and to monitor your sleep at home with a sleep log for a week or two before being evaluated at the center. Next you will be interviewed by a sleep specialist. The specialist will review all this information, as well as your doctor's summary of your health history. On the basis of your questionnaire, sleep log, interview, and health history, the center's professional team will decide whether you need to sleep overnight in the laboratory.

In most cases a person with insomnia will be asked to sleep in the lab only if there is evidence to suspect a medical cause of the insomnia. Otherwise, the specialist will use the information you provided to give you recommendations for improving the quality of sleep. The specialist also may refer you to a physician or psychologist experienced in helping insomnia sufferers learn to sleep better.

WHAT HAPPENS IN THE SLEEP LAB

If you sleep overnight in the lab, someone from the sleep disorders center will give you guidelines telling how to prepare for your stay. The instructions typically include these:

- *Don't nap during the day before you sleep at the lab.*

- *Don't use alcohol for twenty-four hours before you go to the lab.*

- *Don't take caffeine in any form after breakfast on the day you go to the lab.*

- *Eat a regular evening meal before you go to the lab.*

- *Bring nightclothes, a robe, slippers, and any personal hygiene items you may need.*

If you regularly use any type of medication, ask the center staff if you should take it that day. In most cases, you will be told to avoid sleep medication, sedatives, and antidepressants for two weeks before being evaluated. Talk to the prescribing physician if there is a possibility of problems with drug withdrawal during this period.

At the center, a technician will show you around and help you feel at ease. Every sleep disorders center contains two adjacent rooms. The technician remains in the control room all night, monitoring measurements from your body. An intercom permits you to talk to the technician from your bed in the next room, which often is set up like a typical home bedroom.

After you are ready for bed, the technician will use glue or tape to attach several electrodes — small flat metal disks — to the surface of your head. Electrodes placed on the scalp record electrical impulses the brain emits as signals to the rest of the body. These impulses, caused by the firing of the brain's hundred billion nerve cells, are called brain waves. Brain waves are the object of most interest to sleep researchers. The record from the scalp electrodes, measuring these brain waves, is called an electroencephalogram (EEG).

In addition, electrodes are usually attached to the temples to record eye movements and to the chin to record muscle tension. Sensors can be placed in front of your nostrils to measure the temperature and flow of your breathing. Bands around your abdomen and chest measure breathing movement. Electrodes attached to your legs measure whether your legs twitch during sleep. Electrodes on your chest record data about your heart function.

You may be wondering how anyone can possibly fall asleep when covered with electrodes and lying in a strange bed. In fact, people rarely have difficulty sleeping in the lab. Most patients quickly become accustomed to the wires and electrodes. The technician can unplug them easily if the person needs to get out of bed during the night.

Many insomnia sufferers actually sleep *better* in the lab than at home. People with conditioned insomnia (Chapter 12) sleep better in unfamiliar environments than in their own beds. Other people feel relieved that a team of professionals is taking their insomnia seriously, and this positive feeling helps induce sleep. Don't worry that you may not sleep well in the lab. If you can't sleep, your sleeplessness will give the team at the sleep disorders center information to study and analyze.

The electrodes and sensors on your body are connected to a *polysomnograph* in the control room. This is a machine that records measurements from your sleeping body. A computer or a technician then converts the data to a somnogram like the one on page 35.

The next day, a physician or psychologist will examine and interpret the data. This sleep specialist will see how long it took you to fall asleep, how you progressed through the different sleep stages, and whether you showed signs of irregular breathing, leg movements, or other physical problems. Then you will meet with the specialist to discuss your sleep and how you can improve it.

Index